PRE-MED HANDBOOK

PRE-MED
HANDBOOK

Howard Levitin, M.D.

WARNER BOOKS

A Warner Communications Company

Copyright © 1986 by Howard Levitin
All rights reserved.
Warner Books, Inc., 666 Fifth Avenue, New York, NY 10103

W A Warner Communications Company

Printed in the United States of America
First Printing: April 1986
10 9 8 7 6 5 4 3 2 1

Library of Congress Cataloging-in-Publication Data

Levitin, Howard.
  Pre-med handbook.

  1. Medical colleges—Admission. 2. Medicine—
Vocational guidance. 3. Medical colleges—United States
—Directories. 4. Medical Colleges—Canada—
—Directories. I. Title. [DNLM: 1. Education, Medical—
United States. 2. Education, Premedical—United States.
3. Educational Measurement. 4. Schools, Medical—
Canada—directories. 5. Schools, Medical—United
States—directories. 6. Students, Premedical.
W 18 L666P]
R838.4.L48 1986   610'.7'1173   85-18004

ISBN 0–446–38291–4 (U.S.A) (pbk.)
      0–446–38292–2 (Canada) (pbk.)

Book design: *H. Roberts Design*

To David and Amy, the "dynamic duo"
who make it all worthwhile
and
To the memory of Joan,
who made a remarkable contribution to
my well-being and remains a continuing inspiration.

ACKNOWLEDGMENTS

Many hands and minds contributed to this book—but only a few are noted here. To those who helped in small and unknown ways we owe our deep appreciation and thanks.

Without Jeffrey Weiss's encouragement, the *Pre-med Handbook* would never have appeared. In the early days he shepherded it to publishers, making sure that it landed safely in the right hands at Warner Books. To him our first bow, especially for his generosity and kindness.

Similarly, Seymour Ubell played a key role. His support smoothed out obstacles that would have stood in the way, making it far more difficult to accomplish. Our gratitude for his steadfast commitment.

Designer Rudi Wolff provided his sensitive and sophisticated talents. Tom Repensek, whose care and attention to minute details will surely be appreciated by all those who study the data, created the directory of U.S. and Canadian medical schools. Elaine Cacciarelli helped in many ways, not least by her patience, but also by reviewing parts of the manuscript. Barbara Alpern and Laureen Scimeca provided consistently efficient, accurate, and handsomely typed manuscripts.

Laurence J. Kirshbaum, president of Warner Books, who immediately grasped the importance of this project, cleared the way with dispatch, permitting complete freedom and providing every support. Equally, our editor, Patti Breitman, was consistently enthusiastic and resourceful. To her and to unseen hands at work at Warner, we offer our thanks.

My daughters Jennifer and Elizabeth are singled out—for their love and especially to let them know how much I love them. Rosalyn Deutsche, who provided comfort and concern, will never know how much she contributed.

—*Robert Ubell, Executive Editor*

I wish to thank Pamela Nyiri, Director of Financial Aid at the Yale School of Medicine, for assistance in preparing and reviewing the Financial Aid section; and Janet Pickett for her patience and skill with word processing.

I especially want to thank Robert Ubell, who introduced me to and guided me through the demanding world of publishing. His expertise and patience were much appreciated.

—*Howard Levitin, M.D.*

NOTICE

The information contained in the directory section of U.S. and Canadian medical schools was provided in the summer of 1985 by those schools listed and reflects the data provided by the schools at that time. Every effort has been made to publish the most up-to-date and accurate information. Note, however, that all the data, as they appear here, are subject to change. Nothing in the directory or the rest of this book is binding on the schools listed, the author, or Warner Books. Information about nine schools listed—the University of California San Diego School of Medicine, Indiana University School of Medicine, University of Minnesota Medical School at Minneapolis, University of New Mexico School of Medicine, East Carolina School of Medicine, Temple University School of Medicine, Northwestern University Medical School, University of Iowa College of Medicine, and University of

Arizona College of Medicine—is derived from public records. These nine schools did not provide information for the directory in this book.

Before applying to any school listed, students should contact the school directly to obtain the most recent and accurate information.

Nothing is this book shall be construed as a guarantee to admit applicants to any medical school in the U.S. or abroad.

CONTENTS

7. Rejection

8. Your Finances

9. Directory of U.S. and Canadian Medical Schools

Preface:
Are You
Considering A
Medical Career?

Before committing yourself to medicine, a life you know about only vaguely, it would be good to take some hours and curl up with this book. You need not read it page by page, as if it were a novel or a textbook on which you will be tested tomorrow morning. Some chapters may apply to your life—others may be irrelevant. So skip those parts that you think won't be of much help.

But I urge you to take a close look at certain important sections—even if you think you know all about them already. Read, especially, the chapters about your own life and motivation. You'll be surprised to discover how much you can learn about yourself and why you're thinking about becoming a doctor.

And don't skip the chapters about what it will be like to be a doctor when you graduate. If you read nothing else before you apply to medical school, the sections on the future doctor's life should be required. There are lots of misconceptions about being a physician today, and very few people know what is in store for those who will practice in the next decades. Since you're likely to devote most of your life to your work as a doctor—if you succeed in getting into medical school—it's wise to know ahead of time what you're getting yourself into.

No doubt, you've absorbed a great deal of information about doctors, their incomes, their lives, from many sources—books, TV, movies, advisers, friends, relatives. Although some of what you've learned may be accurate, a good deal is certainly wrong. And if you're thinking about entering medicine based on a few very shaky facts, it would be best to take a closer look.

Many who have been successful and have been accepted into medical school have been sadly misled into believing that their academic abilities will carry them through all the challenges they will face. Unfortunately, most high schools and colleges reward you with high grades for academic accomplishment and you may feel that those achievements are sufficient. Your teacher may have said, "This is Biology 101. Our textbook has 132 pages in sixteen chapters. Read it and learn it all." If you did well, you may feel that now that you know some facts, you understand what medicine is about.

If you apply and are accepted to medical school, you will discover that the body of knowledge that your professors will ask you to assimilate is not well defined and, shockingly, is virtually unlimited. You may suddenly realize, after your first few years of training, that much of what you learned has been turned around and made obsolete by new and important findings from research. Someone once said, "Continuing medical education is a forced reminder of my perpetual ignorance." Many students cannot cope with uncertainty. It causes them great anxiety, and they often find to their regret that they never should have chosen medicine in the first place.

As a doctor, you will need to cope with something even more troubling than uncertainty: death and dying. Doctors have not always handled this well. And now that patients, their families, and professionals from other spheres are pressuring physicians to look more closely at how they face the facts of life and death, you'll need to examine your own way of dealing with these dramas.

If and when you become a doctor, the world will not be the same. What we know and understand about medical practice today will have little or no bearing on the style and approach you will follow ten years from now. The solo practitioner is already an endangered species, and in all likelihood, you will be working for a salary as a member of a large team. What's more, the future may hold possibilities for practice that never existed before—high technology, ultraspecialization, and a wide landscape of other fascinating, new fields. By the time you become a doctor, there will be careers in medicine totally unknown today.

As a doctor, you'll need many qualities, not the least of which will be reasonable intelligence. But a good mind will not be enough; you'll be called upon to test your intelligence by remembering and putting to practical use a large body of detailed factual knowledge. Computers will surely help to recall and retrieve information, but it will continue to be important for you to *think*.

And while it is overdrawn on TV as an almost every-minute-of-the-day drama, you undoubtedly are aware that occasionally you will be called upon to make life-and-death decisions. This awesome responsibility is carried by every doctor every day of his or her life.

As a doctor, you'll discover that little is certain in medicine. In some cases neither your books nor your colleagues will be of help. A good doctor learns to cope honestly with uncertainty yet retain the patient's confidence.

Despite spectacular advances in medical technology and basic science, doubt still persists. Yet today patients are wiser about medical uncertainty than ever before, and as people become more involved and knowledgeable about their own health, they will begin to share more in decisions about their own treatment. Patient involvement relieves doctors of some of the anxiety and pressure they feel when left to make decisions alone. By the time you become a doctor (if you decide to be one), this change in medical care may turn out to be one of the great advances of the century. If you expect to act as a high medical priest, tending to your patient flock with all the power and control that comes with practicing traditional medicine, you should be aware that change is on its way. Chances are, you will never exert such commanding authority when you become a doctor.

Medical care financing is now undergoing such dramatic change that by the time you are a doctor, who pays for health care, how it's paid, and how much may be altogether different from costs and arrangements made today. Government, health-insurance companies, and patients are all pressuring for lower medical costs. Doctors, who until now have been viewed as distinguished members of society, contributing to its welfare, may be seen in the future as merely another actor in the health-care business.

Many believe that we already have more physicians

than are needed. Some reports predict that by the year 2000 there will be a "glut" of doctors in the U.S. Whether or not this is true, educators and others are beginning to think about decreasing the number of students admitted to medical school and are contemplating cutting back on the number of students in programs leading to medical specialization. If those who say that there are more than enough doctors are right, then your freedom to locate your practice where you'd like will be severely limited. What's more, you can expect to have fewer patients, since there may not be enough to go around. There's a chance that your future income and life-style may suffer.

Added to the possible oversupply of doctors is the introduction of new health-care professionals. Nurse practitioners, nurse midwives, and physician associates are well-trained people with a genuine commitment to deliver good medical care. They may be competing with the future doctor for patients. What's more, they provide patients with a different style of care. Trained as primary-care professionals, they are committed to educating and involving patients in reaching decisions important to their health care. If they emerge as a major force when you practice, your central role will be eroded. Apart from the competition for patients, you may also be faced with competition for the respect and loyalty of your patients.

With corporations entering medicine many physicians now work nine to five as wage earners in large, commercially run facilities. When you become a doctor, there's a good chance that corporations will play an even bigger part in delivering medical care. Corporate medicine will certainly affect the way in which you will practice.

Not surprisingly, science still remains the basis of medical education. After all, modern medicine is based on a solid scientific foundation. So it would be wise for you to take two years of chemistry, a year of biology, and another year of physics, because virtually all medical schools require them. Other science courses have become somewhat less essential.

You need no longer carry bedpans as substantive evidence that you are committed to helping other people. But activities that reflect your interpersonal skills—your desire to be generous, kind, and compassionate—are important. So if you really are genuine about the welfare of others, show your motivation by choosing a caring activity that makes sense for you.

For the applicant it can be both reassuring—and frustrating—to realize how much getting into medical school is a game. Subjectivity—the way a particular interviewer at a particular school looks at you and your record—and just plain luck often play key roles in who gets in and who doesn't.

Medicine is a noble, highly regarded, rewarding profession—and will no doubt remain so, even when you graduate from medical school. But before you apply, understand what it's all about. One of the ways of knowing what you're in for is by reading this book.

1.
Your Life

Is Medicine for You?

The medical profession offers intelligent and highly motivated individuals the opportunity to pursue a rewarding
career, so many highly qualified applicants seek admission
to medical school every year. Yet those of us who have
worked with students have come to realize that too often
the decision to enter medical school was based on an
inadequate perception of what the profession is really like.
Many suffer emotional trauma when they suddenly discover what the real world of medical school and medicine is
all about. While the number of those who abandon medicine midway is not terribly large, those who leave often do
so because they recognize, a little too late, that medicine
was not a wise emotional choice for them.

Your Intellectual Skills

Rarely do students find that they are unable to meet the intellectual challenges. Most are quite well prepared for the long hours of study, the requirement to absorb large quantities of information, the assimilation of strange and confusing new jargon, and the understanding of complex scientific theories and evidence.

Very likely, if you are admitted, you will be well prepared for the intellectual life of medical school. And it should be no surprise, because if you do get in, you already will have leapt over the intellectual hurdles that stood in your way on the path leading to medical school. If you are like nearly all students who are admitted, you will have earned an academic record at college that was somewhat above average. You also will have performed well in other ways that showed your intellectual skills. There is a very good chance that you worked very hard to achieve your status and the command of your subjects. If you earned a prominent record as an undergraduate, you will be able to manage in medical school when you are confronted by similar, but more demanding, tasks. They will require the very same qualities you already possess—perseverance, industry, and intelligence.

Are You Emotionally Prepared?

While you may be intellectually equipped, you may not have the emotional resources to persevere. It would be wise for you to consider who you are and whether you are up to taking on the psychologically taxing challenges ahead. Many find that they do not possess the strengths required, and so it would be best if they turned to other professions. Others learn that their personalities seem to fit quite well with medicine, and so they go on to become fine doctors.

The old joke goes: If you can't stand the sight of blood, you'd better not be a doctor. While it's not too funny, there's still some truth in it. And the same goes for other things that are part of a physician's world. Death, for instance. How good are you at coping with it? Some people do not handle it terribly well. They can fall into deep mourning for long periods. Others, luckily, have the capacity to integrate it into their emotional lives and are able to deal with its profound effects on themselves and other people. Some turn away altogether, never permitting it to affect them—or at least not consciously admitting that it touches them. Some people—perhaps yourself— have never really thought about it or considered what effect it might have on them. But since death will surely confront you often as a doctor, it is important to give it some thought now and consider whether you will be able to come to terms with it as a routine part of your professional life.

Death is only one of a number of troubling things that will face you in medical school and, later, when you practice. For example, how good are you at sharing the intimacies of other people's personal lives? Would it seriously disturb you to learn about a patient's sexual activity? Would you feel free to encourage your patients to talk about themselves? Based on your relationships with your family, friends, and fellow students, you already know how good you are at listening to others, how much at ease you are in gaining other people's confidence, how generous you are in offering support and comfort. Look yourself in the eye: Are you the kind of person who finds it relatively easy to interact with others, or is contact with others a strain?

In medical school, by and large, students learn to overcome their embarrassments and timidity at observing naked patients. With time they adjust to these situations. But it's important to ask yourself now: Will you be able to learn to act with dignity and maturity when the time comes?

If you are easily thrown by unusual events; if things tend to cause you serious anxiety; if you are quick to anger; if you are generally uneasy with people—think twice and then once again about a medical career. You'll be confronted with so many obstacles in medical school and later in your practice that it would be unwise for you to go on.

But, if after thinking hard about these important emotional considerations, you still feel you can handle them, there's a very good chance you will. Students admit that life in medical school is not easy, that they are threatened by its emotional demands, but most have survived and, miraculously, blossomed.

For many of those who eagerly look forward to medical school, timidity, emotional turmoil, and embarrassment are not serious problems. Most students considering a career in medicine recognize their strengths, and for most, their interpersonal skills are in part what made them think about becoming a doctor in the first place.

At the other end of the emotional spectrum, however, are those who think a little too highly of their abilities. In fact, the determination required to achieve on so many fronts and to persevere under competitive conditions can shape the kind of personality that is often detrimental to patients. With luck medical school admissions committees will spot these students and screen them out. But you know yourself better than any committee member, better than any interviewer. Look deeply into your soul: Would it be better for you to turn to law or finance where your driving, intense qualities might be better suited? Remember that you will be treating frightened, vulnerable patients who will need your compassion. No doubt you've passed many academic tests with high honors, but can you be humble and humane—the most important test?

Remember, too, that the era of the commanding, authoritative physician is coming to a close. Your position will be challenged not only by hospital administrators, corporate health managers, government regulators, and others in power, but also by newly emerging actors on the medical stage—the nurse practitioner, the physician assistant, and other allied health professionals. And your patients, above all, mostly subtly but sometimes overtly, will demand that you share medical decisions with them. So if you're the kind of person who seeks advice from others, who feels comfortable sharing decisions, who is stimulated by collaborative efforts—the future of medicine is with you. But if you'd rather stick to the old medical priesthood tradition, with decision-making power resting exclusively with you, a medical career in the last decades of this century is not likely to make you happy.

You also won't be happy if you need certainty. Often doctors make decisions based on very shaky evidence. Before you fill out your first medical-school application form, ask yourself: "Do I need to be reassured that everything I do is *correct*? Do I need to remove all doubt before making a decision?" In medicine there is often no consensus. Sometimes good doctors learn that their judgment turns out to be ill-advised, even after long and difficult investigation. If you cannot accept this kind of failure, success in medicine will elude you.

Success and Money

There is no denying that in our society success often equals money. And since we all know that doctors tend to make a lot of money, they are certainly among the most "successful." When you become a doctor, you'll surely earn more than the average American, so there's a good chance you will succeed—if money is your goal. But you can also make a good deal of money in finance, management, and many other professions. For those looking to medicine principally as a way of earning large sums of money, it does not appear to be a wise career choice. You will be spending many years at considerable expense, concentrating your attention on anatomy, physiology, biochemistry, and other difficult subjects, when you could more profitably spend your time and your resources studying the market, banking, or more productive financial areas designed expressly to build fortunes.

In the coming decades medicine will be less lucrative. As government and insurance companies force doctors to reduce costs, as corporations assume larger responsibilities for health-care delivery and employ more physicians on salary, and as other pressures ultimately come to reduce the doctor's income, chances are good that your earnings as a physician practicing in the 1990s will be a good deal less than what most doctors have come to expect.

As a doctor, you'll surely live a comfortable, perhaps even a privileged life, even as the profession's income shrinks. But if medicine appeals to you principally because of its income possibilities, it might be best if you looked elsewhere.

Pre-med Syndrome

Now that you've weighed yourself on your emotional and intellectual scales and you've decided that medicine is attractive and your qualities fit it well, you now must decide something equally important. Will your participation in the race to get into medical school be based exclusively on your achievements—or will you fall victim to a disease among undergraduates, known as the "pre-med syndrome"? It afflicts large numbers of students and unleashes some of the most unscrupulous acts and characteristics in the people it attacks—cheating on exams, failing to cooperate with other students, and falsifying credentials.

Of course, the choice is yours. You can succumb to the pre-med syndrome or you can resist it. Chances are good that if you succumb to the hysteria and the fierce competition, you may not get into medical school. The disease is easily spread from student to student, and its signs are often obvious to admissions committees and interviewers.

The admissions process is very carefully monitored for error and falsification, so take great care in preparing your application. Even if you haven't come down with the pre-med syndrome, remember that an innocent error may be misinterpreted as a form of deception.

The pre-med syndrome has one other serious side effect. Often undergraduates apply to medical school as if it were a big-game sport, with the trophy being acceptance. Many students fall into it without recognizing that their desire to get into medical school has been propelled by their friends and fellow students who are in a fury to win the race. If everybody is so keen to get in, why aren't you? Try to resist if you find that you've just fallen in with the pace.

Is Medicine for You or for Your Parents?

And now the very last question before you apply: Are you considering medical school based on your own desires, or are you under parental pressure? Often this is the most difficult question to answer, because most people cannot easily unravel what they expect of themselves and what their parents expect of them. This is especially true for students who set medical school as a goal when they are quite young. Still, this may be the right moment to think about it and try to determine who wants you to get into medical school—you or your parents?

Remember that your parents will not be spending the next eight years working harder than they ever have in their lives. Their disappointment, if you decide against medical school, will be of a much shorter duration.

A Final Word to Parents and Students

There is a common conversation that takes place at home, and it goes something like this: "What are you planning for your career?" Response: "Not sure yet." Query: "It's your third year in college. You must decide." Response: "I will." Query: "Have you decided for or against medicine?" Response: "I'm not sure." Quote from parents: "You should decide for yourself. We do not want to pressure you."

But let's face it: In a good number of cases this final statement is either false or meaningless. Parental pressure is felt, even when denied. Children learn early what their parents expect them to accomplish, and parents let it be known—quietly or aggressively—what careers they feel are most desirable. Children know that falling short causes disappointment.

A lifetime of encouragement cannot be erased simply by saying "We do not wish to pressure you." Children feel the pressure that parents exert, even when expressed silently. It may be best for both parents and children to enter a dialogue to state preferences openly, rather than having parents pretend that they do not care about the choices made by their children. It's wise not to try to make bright children think that it doesn't matter one way or the other.

Students certainly owe their parents a great deal. As a matter of basic courtesy, they should participate civilly in discussions about their future. But even though you owe your parents a lot, try not to pay them back by accepting a lifetime of misery in a career you never wanted.

2.
A Doctor's
Life

The Changing Medical Profession

Our perception of the medical profession in general, and the doctor's role in particular, has undergone dramatic change. In the twenty-five to thirty years since the end of the Second World War and up until the 1970s, the physician was held in high regard, respected, even revered: a pillar of the community, an esteemed citizen. This was true in spite of the fact that the physician's ability to understand and cure disease was fairly limited. For the most part doctors could only stand by in a supportive role for their patients as the natural course of medical events unfolded.

Yet during this very period medicine's ability to understand and cure disease has improved dramatically. Witness the eradication of polio and tuberculosis or our ability to understand genetic diseases; the introduction of organ transplantation, laser therapy, CAT scanning, and a broad range of other therapies and diagnostic techniques.

Ironically, just as the power of medicine has expanded, the status of the physician has declined. Today doctors are in the unenviable position of being seen by the public as entrepreneurs, businessmen concerned more with cash flow, investment, and profit margins than they are with the care of their patients. Why has this happened? Commentators explain this shift by pointing to many causes. And, no doubt, no one explanation is correct.

This trend is not unique to medicine. All institutions are now being questioned. No section of society—neither government nor business, nor the professions or labor unions—is exempt. Perhaps because we expect physicians to act at the highest levels of conduct, doctors are more vulnerable to scrutiny. As an aspiring candidate to the medical profession, it is crucial that you are aware of these changes. It is essential that you recognize that the respect once given to doctors and the life-style they enjoyed as a consequence are steadily eroding.

Older medical practitioners commonly say, "I am my own boss. I am totally independent." While this has been true for many doctors, young physicians entering practice will not find it so any longer. With relentless persistence government, industry, and other forces and institutions have altered the pattern. Few doctors can act on their own. Rules and regulations must be followed. Medical fees are set by government, insurance companies, and others. Medicare and Medicaid demand conformity to preset principles. New and untested systems, such as Diagnostic Related Groups, dictate what laboratory tests patients are privileged to have.

Let us look at some of the factors contributing to these changes.

Accountability

No longer free to exert unlimited authority, institutions are now being held more accountable for their actions. In response the medical profession has undergone vast changes. Physicians must now answer to many other actors on the great medical stage: local, state, and federal governments; insurance companies; their fellow doctors; and perhaps most important, their patients.

The dramatic increase in the number of malpractice suits and malpractice costs is not caused, in my opinion, by the sudden revelation of blatantly bad practice. Rather, it is caused by the demand—new to the profession—by patients to become involved in their own medical care. Patients now, as never before, require explanation, participation, and evidence of genuine concern for their well-being. These new demands are created by patients who perhaps reject cold and callous high technology. Perhaps patients have become disillusioned and distrustful of a doctor's concern. Whatever the reasons, patients want and expect to receive something more than proper, up-to-date medical care.

High Cost of Medical Care

Certainly a prime factor in reassessing the medical profession is the high cost of medical care, often inappropriately attributed exclusively to the physician's desire to make a lot of money. These spiraling costs have emerged as an inevitable result of the introduction of remarkable new technologies, accompanied by greed. While physicians cannot be exonerated, they cannot, and should not, be held totally responsible.

Nonetheless, physicians have failed to be sensitive to the needs of their patients. They have largely assumed that since modern medicine is better than ever, their interpersonal skills and compassion are perhaps less important.

Life-styles and Styles of Practice

Many physicians, swept up in the new narcissism—the "me generation"—have focused more of their attention on their own life-styles and financial rewards. Traditionally, in return for respect and prestige physicians frequently responded with dedication and commitment. Today physicians graduating in the 1980s often are more concerned than ever with the good life and high income.

These days, students entering their postgraduate training seek out those programs where the hours are good, rather than where the training may be superior. Those residency programs demanding every-other-night "on-call" schedules are far less popular (in spite of the prestige attached to them) than those with lighter requirements. Salary is also an important factor in students' choices, as is the location and the cultural environment. Long gone is the intern of the 1950s who worked around the clock for as little as twenty-five dollars a month—and sometimes at no salary at all. It should come as no surprise then that as we accept these attitudes, the doctor-patient relationship undergoes dramatic change.

It would have been unheard of twenty-five years ago for an obstetrician to tell *his* (most physicians were male then) patient that his practice consists of himself and his three colleagues who work together in group practice. Today, most obstetricians assure their patients that one of the doctors in the group will be on call and in attendance when she goes into labor.

Most patients nowadays do not assume that their own doctor will be there: Traditional personal attention is neither offered nor expected. Consequently it is no coincidence that recent graduates have deluged obstetrical programs in unprecedented numbers. Similarly other well-paying (but, according to students, not the reason), better life-style specialties are attracting larger numbers of graduates. Ophthalmology, ear-nose-and-throat, dermatology, and radiology are high on the list.

Solo practice, for a small, defined patient population, where the doctor goes on house calls, is essentially gone. Group practice, with two or more physicians—usually four to a group—is very popular. There is every reason to expect that these will continue to flourish.

Large group practices, corporations with physicians as shareholders, and medical conglomerates, such as the Kaiser Foundation, Humana, and Hospital Corporation of America are flourishing, and others loom on the horizon. These large-scale health-care organizations will offer attractive financial and life-style packages to young physicians. And large corporations, troubled by the rising cost of prepaid health insurance for their workers, are likely to hire physicians to render health care to their employees.

Compassion and Ethical Behavior

Also emerging in the health-care system is the new health professional—the physician assistant, nurse practitioner, midwife, and others—who are well-trained and able to play an important role in the delivery of health care. These new medical workers have carved out another niche in the traditional doctor-patient relationship. They have been introduced, in part, to offer patients more caring and personalized health-care services.

Medical educators are aware and concerned, recognizing that the trend toward high-technology diagnosis and treatment, team care, and other factors are leading health care down the road toward further depersonalization. In response, medical schools are being asked to enroll more compassionate and humane students, hoping to graduate physicians who care more for their patients. To this end medical schools are also urged to broaden their curricula to include humanities, social science, and ethics.

While I have no argument with these noble efforts, I fail to see how we can modify behavior by offering courses in literature and ethics. As in the past, students will fulfill society's expectations and will follow the lead of their role models—their parents, teachers, and practicing physicians. For example, as a medical student, you no doubt will learn about cost containment. You will be exhorted to use your best efforts to reduce your patient's and the nation's medical bills. From the classroom you will go to a hospital as an apprentice, and you will discover that cost containment is often disregarded. *Ethics* can be taught as a formal course, but *ethical behavior* must be demonstrated. Learning about the humanities does not make you more humane.

Patients' Rights and Public Awareness

Historians will speak of the 1980s as the period when patients claimed their medical rights. As patients tend to diminish their respect for their physicians, they also tend to lose their trust in the profession. Patients may wonder, "Is my doctor doing this for me or for money?" Insurance companies, for example, have begun to advise and often require their subscribers to seek a second opinion before agreeing to surgery or expensive, high-technology procedures. Reports show that when a second opinion is obtained, a significant percentage of initially recommended procedures are found to be unnecessary. It is no wonder that many patients now question their physician's motives.

People are also far more knowledgeable about medicine than ever before. Newspapers, radio, television, and magazines deluge us with medical information. Syndicated "Ask Your Doctor" columns appear everywhere. Radio and TV news programs offer special segments by "your health and medicine reporter." Cable television broadcasts twenty-four-hour health channels. Even programs designed especially for physicians are aired publicly and seen by nonprofessionals. Magazines and newsletters exclusively devoted to health care and prevention are widely read. News stories and information about smoking, drinking, the environment, and safety all contribute to an unprecedentedly informed public. Physicians even joke about the fact that they learn about the latest medical "breakthrough" from the newspaper, long before their medical journal arrives.

History will judge whether all this public awareness and concentration on health is good or bad for us. Nevertheless, it is a fact and has become an important part of the physician-patient exchange. When your patient says, "But, doctor, I read that . . . ," there is no doubt that your authority is undermined, however unintentionally. As a doctor, you will be called upon to acknowledge this challenge to your authority and to cope with it.

Authority and Decision-making

If part of your desire to practice medicine includes your wish to control the medical destiny of your patients and to play an authoritarian role, you should be aware that things are changing. The doctor no longer makes all the decisions. High technology, and its associated high cost, has forced decisions about its use and value out of the closed physician's club and into wide public debate. Other medical issues are no longer exclusively in the hands of doctors. The use of life-support systems in the face of unlikely recovery, transplantation (especially animal to human), artificial organs, genetic engineering, and the nature and origin of life itself command national attention. In the midst of this turmoil the fundamental question emerges: Who decides the medical destiny of a particular patient?

While the traditional high-priest physician dealing with a supplicant patient is fading, many patients still prefer to give their doctors exclusive responsibility for medical decisions. Patients challenging decisions made by their physicians can express distrust and lack of confidence. Often, troubled patients do not want to jeopardize their treatment or undermine someone who plays such a significant part in their lives.

But people are rapidly becoming aware that trust and confidence alone are not the issue. Many know that modern medical competence, remarkable as it is, has its limits. Decisions are not always clear-cut or scientifically sound. Treatment is often based on judgment, not so much on undeniable fact. Judgment is open to interpretation. Interpretation can often depend on questions having little to do with medicine and a lot to do with wishes, needs, and values.

Consider what happens when a patient is diagnosed as having pneumonia, caused by the common pneumococcus bacteria. The decision as to how to best treat the patient is subjected to a standard process that ultimately comes down to: "What if I do?" versus "What if I don't?" In this case the answer is easy because it does not carry the weight of moral or value judgments: Treating the disease with penicillin carries an extremely low risk, and withholding therapy can seriously endanger the patient's life. With penicillin recovery is expected to be complete, with no thought given to the chance of an impaired post-therapy life-style. The decision is easy, and consequently, patients are rarely consulted about the choice because it is obvious and there is little risk.

But today decisions often are not so simple. Frequently they include considerations not only about life and death, but also about quality of life, cost, and other critical factors. In this environment physicians must enter a new style of dialogue with their patients.

Leaving aside those rare physicians who base their

decisions on financial gain or their need to exercise their authority, how can genuinely concerned physicians offer their *best* advice? But the question is: Best for whom? As a doctor, would it be good to imagine, "If I were in my patient's shoes, what would I do?" and then recommend a course of action? In my view this approach is well intentioned but inappropriate. Your values are your own; they may be quite different from your patient's.

Consider surgery versus medical management for a life-threatening disease. It may be a choice between open-heart surgery or drug treatment for coronary heart disease. Or it may be a high-risk surgical procedure to remove a malignant tumor as opposed to chemotherapy. These choices may include questions of risk of survival and damaging the quality of life—perhaps with serious physical limitations, impotence, and reduced intellectual productivity. Clearly such decisions must be made by the patient. The degree to which a sedentary life, sexual inadequacy, or diminished mental capacity is acceptable or terrifying depends on each patient's own emotional response.

"But," says the skeptic, "good physicians know their patients so well that they are able to take all these issues into consideration." Nonsense. No one can know all of the intimate details of another person's inner thoughts, anxieties, and aspirations and be able to place themselves in their shoes.

"But patients are not M.D.s and cannot make these decisions. They do not know enough." Even more nonsense. Doctors often use this argument to avoid the emotional commitment and time it takes to *help* their patients through these crises. Of course, patients do not become medically knowledgeable suddenly. The wise doctor outlines the risks, complications, and medical facts that apply. With this knowledge the patient can choose intelligently.

Some respond, "I do not want to get involved. I trust my physician and I prefer that he or she decide." Of course, such patients must be respected, even though their reluctance may be based on traditional doctor-patient relationships.

Occasionally physicians treat their patients as submissive recipients of their medical dictates, and suddenly, in the moment of crisis they say, "Okay, you decide." Good medical practice calls for patients to be told at their first meeting with their physician that they will be an involved participant in the ongoing mutual effort to prevent and cure disease, and this, I believe, will become the accepted pattern. With this goal in mind the patient expects to be called upon for decisions and is well prepared emotionally and well informed when the time comes. What's more, compliance with a therapeutic regimen is clearly better when patients understand what is going on, have realistic insights into what can (and cannot) be accomplished, and most importantly, are involved in planning their program. Patients can and should be trusted. After all, they have a vested interest in the outcome.

"Where Will I Practice?"

In the years ahead—if you are lucky enough to become a physician—you will be faced with a basic question. You will ask yourself, "Where would I like to practice?" Yet conditions in the world of medicine will force you to reformulate that question. You may be asking, instead,

"Where will it be possible for me to practice?" What's more, another question may be raised: "Where will I be needed?"

Not too long ago a major study predicted that by the year 1990, the U.S. would have a surplus of physicians. And, by the year 2000, there would be a glut. The report used a number of variables to reach its conclusions: the number of physicians now in practice (adjusted for mortality rates); the number in postgraduate training; the number of students enrolled in medical schools; plus those anticipated to enter medical school over the next twenty years. Using these figures, the study published its conclusions.

Missing, however, was a judgment about how much health care our society wants and is willing to pay for. Look at it this way: It is simple enough to calculate and report, "I have two workers, three shovels, and a wheelbarrow." And then ask, "Do I have the resources to dig a hole?" Well, the answer is, obviously, "Yes and no." Unknown is the size of the hole, the deadline for completion, and instructions on where the excavated dirt should be placed—nearby or at a considerable distance?

Similarly the fundamental question in medical care is: What constitutes *enough* physicians? Surely if every citizen expected a daily medical checkup before embarking on the day's activities, we would be woefully short of physicians. Alternatively, if health care is to be made available only to those who can afford to pay for it (and no health insurance is available), then we already have a glut and it will get worse. Economic and political forces will determine how much society is willing to contribute to the nation's health care. Only when we know what we want and what we will pay can we reach any conclusions about how many physicians are needed. The ratio of one doctor for a specified number of people is a simplistic answer since it fails to address the real questions of needs and costs. But if predictions are correct, as a doctor practicing in the 1990s, you'll face some stiff competition.

Health administrators and economists recognize that today medical care is unequally distributed in the U.S. —too many doctors practice in populated, affluent sections of our country and too few in many urban and rural settings. When it comes time to choose, your options for selecting a site to practice may be limited by economic realities. There may be an insufficient number of patients to support your practice in the area you've selected, or government may step in to relocate physicians to solve the maldistribution, blocking your choice.

Are there too many specialists? Most graduates seek postgraduate specialty training and relatively few prefer primary care. Will the options to pursue the specialty of your choice be limited? Very likely. Again, economic reality, government, and large-scale medical conglomerates may join together to limit your access to specialty training.

The Medical-industrial Complex

While the medical profession may wish to avoid facing it, the impact of the medical-industrial complex is already upon us. Large corporate entities, engaged in for-profit medicine, are here. The implications for medicine are enormous. These organizations already employ large numbers of physicians. As they grow they will tend to regulate physicians' hours of practice, control their income, and establish their job relocations, perhaps similar to the way in which executives in industry are shifted around the country.

Good or bad, the medical-industrial complex will not go away. For too long, the medical profession has had its head in the sand, like an ostrich. Remember that the unique anatomical configuration required to place your head in the sand leaves other anatomical locations remarkably vulnerable to assault.

Your Future

These difficulties all seem to offer arguments against going into medicine. Why put yourself through it all? Why spend thousands of dollars, countless hours, and enormous energy and effort? Because, in the end, even with its problems, medicine is a marvelous profession, allowing you to combine your intellectual abilities and your genuine concern for people to do something useful and personally rewarding. These essential components of the practice of medicine will persevere.

But after many years of talking to students in medical school, it is very clear that many were not aware of, or did not give serious thought to, the issues raised here. In the next decades—when you will be practicing, if you are accepted to medical school—these questions are going to become more complicated before they are sorted out. You should know what lies ahead. You'll be better prepared.

Of all the activities you might undertake in college to help you understand what medicine is like, you can do no better than work with a practicing physician. If you can, spend a week or more following him or her around during the working day. Become aware of the day-to-day activities. Overhear the physician-patient dialogue. You'll discover that it is often pleasant, rewarding, and satisfying. But you'll also learn that it can be difficult and frustrating. Discover that the practice of medicine can be very routine, that the exciting melodrama of TV does not occur every moment. Become aware that a surgeon pays the rent not only by treating dramatic cases but also by taking care of patients with varicose veins, hemorrhoids, and infected toenails, that the exciting case of the week may turn out to be a hernia, not open-heart surgery.

If you're lucky, you'll learn that every patient, treated even for minor afflictions, needs your skill and is very grateful. Whatever happens to the medical profession in the years ahead, your patients will still be very important to you. And there's little doubt that you will be very important to them. If your relationship with your patients grows into a fruitful, useful, and productive exchange, it will be because of your attitude and your competence.

There is no question that you can be a competent physician. Your acceptance to medical school indicates that you have the intellectual ability. That you will cultivate those other qualities that will make you a caring, compassionate doctor who treats his or her patients as a partner is up to you.

3.
The
Medical
Student's
Life

What to Expect in Medical School

Medical school is exciting, exhilarating, depressing, frustrating. Before we get to the high points, let's consider some of those frustrations first. Perhaps your first big disappointment will be the sad discovery that your first two years closely resemble your college days. Classrooms, lectures, labs, examinations, even the courses themselves are depressingly similar to those you just left behind. And the most startling shock is that there are *no patients*—or, at best, very limited contact with patients!

"Here I am in medical school," many first-year students think. "I came here to heal the sick, to translate my passionate concern for my fellow human beings into effective health care. Why isn't it happening? Why are there no patients?" You'll soon learn to endure those first years—without treating patients—because what you will be studying will be essential to your future clinical training.

The next expectation dashed is that medical school is not quite the "graduate school" you thought it would be. When most people think of medical school, they place it alongside other graduate schools—as just another step after college on the ladder of higher and higher training.

In physics, for example, students who enter graduate departments start at an already reasonably sophisticated level of achievement obtained as undergraduates. Graduate education offers them the chance to expand and deepen their previous experiences along highly specialized and more sophisticated avenues of study. A physics professor would be shocked if his new graduate students failed to know what an atom was or needed to have the principles of force, levers, and pulleys explained.

Yet in medical school things are much different. Unlike their friends who have gone on to study advanced physics, chemistry, or mathematics, first-year medical students—who even may have taken rather advanced biological sciences courses at college—arrive in medical school to encounter the almost foreign language of medicine and the unknown concepts of disease, terms and ideas that have never before been part of their education. To underscore it the Association of American Medical Colleges calls the four years of medical school "undergraduate medical education." Subsequent residency and training in specialty areas is considered "postgraduate education."

Since 1920—in the aftermath of Abraham Flexner's famous report, which called for a wholesale restructuring of medical training in the United States—and until the 1960s, all American medical students followed a similar regimen. Two years of formal classroom study in the basic sciences were followed by two years of clinical work. In their final year students were finally permitted a small number of electives.

By the mid-1960s, things loosened up somewhat. Students were exposed to clinical experiences earlier, even though basic science continued to dominate the first two years. After decades of pursuing rigidly a strict curriculum, students in the 1960s demanded more "relevance" and more contact with patients. They complained, among other things, that medical school was "dehumanizing." In response, schools offered interdisciplinary classes and some early clinical work.

Recently, traditional courses and conventional discipline have gradually returned, even though many schools still retain traces of the trends that emerged in the mid-1960s. While today's students still continue to find early access to clinical medicine highly desirable, frequently the basic science faculty dismisses these desires. As in the past, professors turn their attention instead to what they feel is the far more important task of having students gain a fundamental appreciation of biomedical science as the first step.

Life and Death

Perhaps the deepest emotional adjustment you'll be forced to make is your encounter with gross anatomy. There you will confront a cadaver, probably for the first time in your life. The "dead body" lying there is a shockingly impersonal assemblage of protoplasm. Students often wonder whether their anatomy course is designed to teach them something about the human body or, rather, is a course offered to instill in them a callous approach to life.

The body on the table may represent a failure of medical practice to you, or you may be suddenly and unexpectedly confronted with your own emotional responses to death, evoked perhaps by some connection with a death of a family member or a friend.

More deeply rooted than your revulsion to the pungent smell of formaldehyde and your occasional intestinal discomfort is your own psychological confrontation with death. Many students have never faced death so closely and have never considered its impact on their emotional lives. You may realize in a flash that you have committed yourself to a career that assumes an awesome responsibility over the lives and deaths of others. What's more, most students may never have considered their own mortality. The anatomy lab may present their first vision of their own deaths.

As you adjust to your initial shock—in the midst, perhaps, of struggling with the approach of your first midterm exams—your conflicts, doubts, and fears are frequently repressed in order to devote your energies to learning facts and just getting through. Some schools try to minimize the impact of the student's initial contact with death by delaying the anatomy classes until later. Others offer support and counseling to help students deal with the unexpected impact.

Basic Science

While anatomy is the most dramatic change in your new life, the medical school faculty that teaches basic science—biochemistry, cell biology, physiology, neurobiology, and other fields—will remind you repeatedly that you will fail to be a good doctor unless you absorb all of the material with which they will overwhelm you. Your inability to absorb the smallest detail of each discipline, you will be warned, will surely result in your causing a worldwide epidemic, so disastrous that it will surpass the worst plagues of the Middle Ages.

Although course and lecture titles in most school catalogs are surprisingly similar, the actual content will vary according to the specific interests of each department or lecturer. You will discover that faculty members unabashedly believe that their very specialized area of knowledge is absolutely crucial to the steady progress of modern medicine. They will go to great lengths to inculcate their students with the key importance of their special expertise.

Since you will be exposed to many instructors during the course of your basic-science education—all of whom are convinced of the fundamental significance of their work—you will be relieved to find that in the end you will have received a rather broad appreciation of biomedical science. No doubt you will then be well prepared to go on to your clinical clerkship, even if you may have missed some of the fine points your more demanding professors insisted you master.

Forced to study amino acid sequences or the details of the genetic code, many frustrated students wonder,

"Why do I have to know all this?" Without this knowledge you could leave medical school to practice "cookbook" medicine. Being a cookbook doctor is easy. When your patient walks into your office and tells you where it hurts, you could thumb through the index of your handy medical guide, and there you'll find a list of symptoms and physical signs. You'll discover that your patient most likely suffers from disease X. Tests and treatment can be uncovered by consulting a standard textbook. Practicing medicine this way requires nothing more than your ability to know the alphabet. You do not need to understand anything else. Cookbook doctors never need to worry about making any new observations or contributing to the advance of medical knowledge. Actually cookbook physicians don't really practice medicine at all.

True physicians are those who understand deeply how normal and diseased cells work, how organs function, and that there is an intimate relationship between drugs, cells, and organs. To a scholarly and investigative doctor the patient becomes a challenge, a "mystery" to be solved. Your patient's well-being will frequently depend on your careful review of the patient's history—by asking critical questions about his or her life and by your scientific analysis of the progress of your treatment.

Clinical Medicine, At Last

Occasionally in your first year, but almost certainly in your second, the door to patient care swings open in a course called "Introduction to Clinical Medicine." It teaches the art of history-taking, the physical examination, analysis of lab tests, and, to varying degrees, the pathophysiology of disease. After you acquire rudimentary skills that enable you to fumble through a history-taking session and to perform a physical exam on your fellow students or on paid volunteers, you finally confront your first real patient in a hospital or a clinic.

As your palms begin to sweat, as your heart beats rapidly and your hands tremble, you won't be much good at chatting casually with your patient or making accurate observations. But your early encounters with real patients—stressful as they surely will be for you—must be experienced and endured. When your anxiety recedes to manageable levels, you'll be able to establish a comfortable relationship with your patients. However, your adaptation to your new role as a physician will not be made any easier when your patient turns into a comedian, sensing your discomfort, or becomes aggressive, challenging your authority.

"What is your problem?" the trembling student asks.

"If I knew, I wouldn't be here!" retorts the would-be comic.

Some students adjust to such confrontations with ease; others find it very difficult. In fact, some students are never at ease with patients, even after long practice.

If there is an art to medicine, it's the physician's ability to put a distressed patient at ease, to impart a sense of confidence even before the doctor knows the solution to the problem the patient presents. Experience is by far the best—if not the only—teacher enabling you to gain your patient's trust.

As your experience in the clinical setting generates confidence you may tend to treat your patients routinely, just as another chore. But your patients will expect you to respond to their need for a high degree of personal involvement and concern. As a good doctor, you should be prepared to give your patients what they need and deserve.

For the novice, performing the physical examination adds new fuel to the already high level of the student's adrenal activity. There stands your undressed and embarrassed patient. Not disturbing enough, to confound things you must remember and perform a long series of complicated maneuvers without revealing your own embarrassment and without poking in the wrong places by mistake.

"Why," you wonder, "is the person going to undress in front of me? Why am I allowed to poke and probe this stranger's body? Why does this patient feel free to tell me about venereal disease, sex, hemorrhoids?"

Obviously these are privileges that our society confers upon physicians and few others. The young doctor does not easily accept this new role. As you become more comfortable you'll learn to adjust to one of the most peculiar medical realities: that total strangers will reveal their most private world and their most intimate parts to you, as if they were as close—or closer—to you as to members of their own family.

And remember, your patients share their intimacies with you in confidence. No part of what you learn is casual gossip or cocktail conversation. Trust is expected without question in the physician-patient relationship. When the covenant is violated, you not only harm your patient but also damage the sense of trust all patients feel for their doctors.

Not often talked about, but ever-present in the minds of most students, is the difficult adjustment to the physical examination, especially when the naked patient is someone the young physician finds attractive. Intellectually most of us believe that we should not allow ourselves to be unnerved by the experience. But despite your best rationalization and despite your best efforts to control them, your feelings are stirred. Experience, coupled with a steadfast commitment to the highest ethical standards, will rapidly assuage your anxiety and allow you to be very comfortable in the role of examiner.

Clinical Clerkship

After you've completed your basic science courses and managed to deal with your first patients, you'll next pass through a series of "clinical clerkships," in which you'll be trained in various medical specialties. You'll be one among four to six students on a ward where you'll spend six to eight weeks at each specialty: medicine, pediatrics, surgery, obstetrics, and psychiatry. You'll be apprenticed to "house officers" under whose guidance you'll now begin to apply your knowledge of basic science and your newly acquired skills to solve real clinical problems. Your house officers and attending physicians will play a central role in your clinical training. At this important point in your education you will make the decision to go along the easy path of practicing cookbook medicine or the more gratifying road of becoming an investigative, scholarly doctor.

A word about "house officers." Until recently, upon leaving medical school, the young doctor's first year of training was called "internship," after which you entered your "residency." Today, the internship has been eliminated, and by modern convention, as you move through the stages of postgraduate education, you will be called a "first-year resident," "second-year resident," and so on. You are a house officer during all levels of training.

In the hospital or clinic you'll be assigned to patients, and you will be expected to question and examine them. You'll be asked to record extensively all your observations, which will form part of your patient's permanent record. You'll also learn how to perform minor procedures: how to draw blood and the like. Worst of all, you'll be asked to do all sorts of menial tasks ("scutwork")—find the X rays... take this specimen to the lab... go to the blood bank... get us some pizza....

And then will come your big moment: presenting your newly assigned patient to the attending physician the following morning during "rounds." Aided by your notes (but mostly from memory), you'll relate, concisely yet completely, the clinical information you've learned about your patient. Eventually you'll become confident and be able to present your patient's case calmly.

The next big challenge—both feared and relished—is the moment when you are asked to discuss your case. The attending physician will turn to you and will want to know *your opinion.* "What do you think is going on? What further tests do you think are necessary? What additional observations should be made? What do you think should be done to treat your patient?"

For the novice, the ultimate reward comes when you are told that your diagnosis and evaluation is "correct." No ceremony, no placing of a wreath on your forehead. Perhaps you'll receive a quiet compliment from a nearby resident. Then comes the swelling of pride with the realization: "I can do it!" You will discover, at the end of this long, often grueling obstacle course, that your entire clinical experience has been aimed at developing your confidence to prepare you for the even more arduous task of being a house officer.

The different clerkships (medicine, pediatrics, obstetrics, surgery, psychiatry) each reflect their own patient populations and the style of medicine practiced in each area. In your medical clerkship you will deal primarily with patients who have serious and complicated illnesses, especially those requiring thoughtful diagnosis and complicated management. In surgery you will treat patients who have already had their diagnosis more definitely established and who will require surgical intervention. Pediatrics, obviously, is limited to diseases of the young. You will be confronted with problems of growth and development, nutrition, and adjustment to society. Your obstetrics and gynecology clerkship will deal with medical problems of pregnancy and the gynecological problems of women. In psychiatry you will see patients from all areas, treating those with behavior disorders. As you move through these disciplines, you will broaden your clinical experience and gain firsthand knowledge, enabling you to appreciate your future choice.

Most medical schools require you to spend some time in an outpatient, ambulatory-care facility where you will observe primary care, the kind of practice that doctors routinely encounter. Your patients will not be so ill as to require hospitalization; nevertheless, they will need diagnosis and management of their medical problems. The kind of relationship you establish with patients in an outpatient clinic is an important component of medical care and ought to be experienced. If your medical school does not offer this opportunity, it could be a disadvantage. It is important to remember that on any given day only five percent of the patients who seek medical care in the United States end up in a hospital. The rest are seen in a wide variety of newly evolving health-care facilities that deliver care to ambulatory patients. Since most physicians will be practicing in this kind of setting, it is essential that you experience it firsthand.

Throughout your clinical apprenticeship on the wards, recurrent questions will float through your mind: "What am I doing here? Do they really know how little I know? Is it fair for me to *practice* on people? What if patients ask questions I cannot answer? Or ask advice I cannot give? Or worse still, ask me if they will die? Should I tell them I'm just a student? Should I fake it? What if a patient takes my advice and it doesn't work? Will it be my fault?"

These and other pounding questions will go through your mind like a looped tape recorder, recurringly demanding answers as you face each new hurdle. Here again, experience will help you cope. Honesty will be good not only for your patient but also for you. It won't help to mislead your patient to believe that you are a world expert. The best thing is to tell your patient that you are a student, that you are learning, but that everything you are doing falls well within the scope of your qualifications and training.

And then comes the moment of truth: the first time one of your patients with whom you have developed a good relationship dies. Your emotional trauma will be multiplied manyfold when death comes to a young patient with great potential and strong family ties. "You did all you could," your friends and supervisors will surely say. They will be very reassuring, but gnawing doubts will remain. Could you have done something more? Should you have read something else? You'll ponder these questions for a long time.

And then other questions will arise: Did the patient know? Was he or she well prepared? What could you have done to increase the patient's comfort? How well prepared was the family? Why was fate so cruel to arrange it so that you would be there and be forced to tell the family? As a young doctor, you'll go through these and other important episodes that will launch you along the road to becoming a competent physician.

You'll also have to face the problem of caring for patients with chronic or incurable diseases. Very likely, such encounters will leave you emotionally drained. You might even wish that the patient would go away. These trials are constant reminders of your inadequacy. Often young physicians create a host of excuses not to go into the room to chat. It is so much easier to say hello to a patient recovering from pneumonia—thanks to miraculous antibiotics—whose only question is, "When can I go home?" than to deal with gnawing and puzzling emotional demands of an incurable patient. You will no doubt learn to bear with it and not abandon your needy cases.

All this talk of death, pain, and sorrow may encourage you to reconsider your decision about medical school. You may think that this section is designed to turn you away from medicine altogether. The reason I have stressed these aspects of your future medical career is that, based on my experience, I have found that students are not well prepared for their emotionally difficult future.

Medicine is—and will remain—a rewarding experience for those who accept the challenge and who recognize their contribution to the welfare of their patients. Your transformation from an eager, young student into a compassionate, sensitive physician, while no easy task, will be a deeply maturing process if you gain insight into what you will face.

"Do I Know All I Have to Know?"

As you wander through the wards you may wonder, "Do I know all I have to know to be a good doctor?" The question is first raised when you're a student. But it doesn't go away, even after years of practicing medicine. It's a chronic cause of anxiety for mature doctors as well as students. With experience, and in time, you'll realize that you'll never know, nor will you ever learn, everything that could be useful to you. There is a small body of knowledge that one must know in order to deal with medical emergencies and urgent situations. You will come to understand, however, that most of the medical information you need to help your patient is available in reference texts and other sources that can be called upon efficiently and effectively.

The real challenge is to know what information you need, how to get it, and to appreciate whether you have the motivation and commitment to take the time and effort to acquire it. Some schools have introduced problem-solving techniques, computers, and other ways to help you find and survey the constantly widening horizon of scientific knowledge. As schools recognize that doctors of the future will be ill-equipped unless they have access to these tools, more of them will begin to offer these new approaches. As your career matures you will realize that patients rarely need immediate solutions to pressing problems. Your treatment will more often depend upon, and benefit from, careful and cautious evaluation. Except in emergency situations, time is on your side.

Making the correct diagnosis is often considered an important first step in providing good health care. True. But keep in mind that many diagnoses are merely descriptive labels, not a statement about the cause of illness. Consider the disease known as disseminated lupus erythematosis. Not uncommonly, physicians diagnose this illness; but still the cause is unknown. It describes a syndrome, or complex set of symptoms, and is useful as a phrase to help physicians communicate with each other. But doctors should not take false pride in having fully diagnosed the disease. The nomenclature for this ailment has its roots in antiquity, when description was all that was available. Patients suffering from the disease have a rash on their faces. To physicians of a bygone era, the rash strongly resembled a wolf's face. Because the red rash tends to be all over the body, doctors came to describe it that way. When translated into ordinary language, disseminated lupus erythematosis means "red wolf disease all over."

Imagine telling your patient, "You have red wolf disease all over." It would hardly instill confidence, let alone be the basis for a legitimate charge for an office visit. Crucial to the maturing process in medicine is the understanding that not only do you have a limited knowledge of many diseases and pathologic processes but also the profession shares your ignorance. Fortunately remarkable progress currently underway in biological science at the cellular and molecular level will rapidly increase our understanding of these previously mysterious diseases to form the basis of future rational therapies.

Electives and Selectives

In your fourth year you'll be offered electives. Some schools provide "selectives," in which you may choose courses from a required group of basic sciences or clinical experiences. Like a Chinese menu, these programs allow you to select one from column A, two from column B, and so on. Certain schools present a broad choice, while others impose strict limits. Still others, while apparently offering great freedom of choice, insist that your selections be approved by tough faculty members or stringent committees.

While electives offer you important opportunities, they are useful only if your choice matches your objectives. Students tend to choose electives for three principal reasons:

1. *"I want to know more about the subject. I really didn't learn enough about it in my earlier courses."* This is the proper pedagogic reason for choosing an elective. It addresses your own self-assessed deficiency and, when successful, is a source of satisfaction. Often students are troubled by this choice because they feel that it may not be in their best interest to expose their ignorance. They fear receiving a poor evaluation and, in the end, diminish their chances for the best postgraduate training. Still, it

takes courage to do what should be done. And it's worth it. But, of course, it may have its price.

2. *"I need to decide on a postgraduate career, and experience in one or more elective will help."* This is an excellent, sound reason. As you work with a surgeon, in the eye clinic, in the cardiac lab, or elsewhere, you'll gain an appreciation of how these specialties work, the intellectual challenges specialists face, and the kinds of patients who seek treatment in these areas. You'll also observe how experienced physicians actually practice in specific types of medical disciplines.

3. *"I need letters of recommendation for my future residency."* This is perhaps the least defensible but regrettably the most common reason for choosing a particular elective. Since it helps play a part in accomplishing their goal, students, not surprisingly, choose those areas where they have already shown competence. Letters of recommendation coming from specialties where students have already proven themselves effective are likely to be flattering.

Most schools allow you to devote some time to electives off campus, at other institutions. You might even choose a location where you think you might like to become a resident. Obviously a good showing at your intended site will enhance your chances of getting a postgraduate position there.

Research

Many schools offer—and frequently encourage—students to undertake a research project, term paper, or other scholarly pursuit. Only one or two schools require a formal dissertation, approved by a committee as a prerequisite to earning a degree. (As of 1985, these schools are Yale and the University of Washington.)

When students participate in quality research, they not only gain valuable firsthand scientific experience, but also they receive a number of other rewards. Of course, on its own, medical research can be pursued as an independent career. It certainly helps to identify your potential interest in research (rather than in a medical practice) by engaging in scientific work. What's more, if a good publication emerges from your research involvement, it can be a valuable addition to your credentials when you apply for postgraduate training.

In-depth study of a particular branch of scientific medicine is valuable for a good many reasons. Apart from helping you build and refine key skills required of all doctors—such as your ability to perform an inquiry successfully and evaluate data—research strengthens your knowledge of concepts of valid scientific procedures and statistical methods. These abilities are likely to play a central role in your life as a physician, whether or not you ever again participate in formal scientific activities.

While most students do not enter a career in research or academic medicine, a high-level medical practice depends on treating your patients as if each one presented you with a research challenge. No physician should ever rest complacently on conventional treatment. Was the therapy that you administered the real cause of the cure? Or did your patient recover simply because the disease continued along its natural path? Knowledge of statistics, chance, and other basic science methods help the good physician to resolve these and other thorny questions.

As a doctor, you'll be overwhelmed with new findings in medical journals, brochures, books, and pharmaceutical advertisements that will deluge your desk. Publishers, learned societies, and drug companies will send you reports that make claims that must be studied and evaluated. Nearly every working day you'll be called upon to make judgments on the value of these claims. Before you accept or reject them, you'll be forced to understand and evaluate them. You'll need to decide their value, based not only on your experience with your patients but also on your knowledge and appreciation of the scientific issues at stake. Your research experience will help you make intelligent assessments of what will come your way.

Evaluations

Just like other academic institutions, medical schools commonly employ examinations, grades, class rank, and other standard ways of measuring your performance. While these criteria are still central, students find that other dimensions of their life are coming under closer scrutiny. Laboratory work, interaction with patients, and other such activities may not weigh as much as "objective" academic scores, but sometimes they do tip the scale.

Your clinical clerkship performance is based primarily on what your attending physician, house staff, and other ward personnel observe and report. Some top students who enter the clinical arena occasionally find that their scholastic edge is blunted by poor evaluations of their clinical work. Others, who may have struggled under the weight of basic science, find that they blossom with patients. The intellectual skill required to master science and the interpersonal finesse needed with patients are complementary and equally important, but as students are stunned to discover, they are quite different. Your college days may have prepared you for the first phase of medical education. Your grade-point average and your MCAT scores can often predict how well you'll do with basic science. But when students are presented with patients, they come up against a challenge for which they are less well prepared. The quiet, shy student often tends to be misinterpreted as uninformed and uninterested. Overly aggressive, pompous, demanding students are not well received, either. (In addition to classroom exams and personal evaluations, many schools also require that students take uniform examinations given by the National Board of Medical Examinations or the Federated State Boards of Medical Examiners.)

Fifth Year (or Leave of Absence for Extended Study)

Many students now extend their studies beyond the traditional four years of medical school. And there are a number of good reasons to take off the year to pursue other avenues. Most medical students have been on an academic treadmill ever since high school. Some feel relieved to be able to jump off for a while, even though they must fight against tremendous peer pressure to continue, since most of their fellow students keep right on going. Most feel that if they stop, they will never accomplish their goals. It is true that some students who take the year off fabricate excuses and avoid doing further serious work, undermining the purpose of their leave.

Perhaps the best reason for taking the break is to do research, to continue work on a project begun, perhaps, as a fourth-year student. Intense involvement in a successful research project can lead to participation in an exciting new discovery and, as mentioned earlier, could provide you with a published scientific paper to add to your academic portfolio.

These days, students who come to medical school are multitalented individuals. Before deciding on medicine, no doubt, many were confronted with the choice of cultivating other pursuits. "Would I have made it in a rock group?" or "Should I have become a computer programmer?" Questions like these persist and sometimes continue to haunt people during the rest of their professional lives.

Some students take the year off to explore careers they may have longed to pursue before they entered medical school. After exposing themselves to their alternative passion, most return to medicine, satisfied that a career as a physician is, after all, their first priority. They return, pleased that they had given themselves one last chance to pursue other desires. These students go back to medicine, happy that their conflicts have been resolved at last. A few, however, realize that the career they had abandoned to enter medical school still holds fascination and attraction. Some never return to medicine. They discover, nearly at the very last minute, that it is not too late to jump off the career express and hop onto another track.

Others who extend their studies do so to complement

their medical training in allied programs in public health, for instance, or in the biological sciences, among other associated studies. Joint-degree programs are becoming rather popular, since they offer students the chance to combine medicine with other fascinating and important areas.

A few students postpone their postgraduate education in order to accompany their spouses or other people with whom they have close relationships (who may be a year behind) into an advanced program. The couple then graduate and go off together for training.

While most schools tend to be quite liberal in granting the extra year of study, you should be aware that some schools ask you to pay additional tuition. Before you decide, consult your school's policy to see if you can manage the year off, especially if it is not tuition-free. The year off may cost you more than you had bargained for.

Getting Help: Advisers and Support Groups

At most schools advisers are available to help students cope with their problems. Advisers may be either full-time or part-time faculty members, clinicians, senior students, psychologists, staff members drawn from the office of student affairs, or others who help students adjust to the rigors and anxieties of medical school. Some advisers are available to talk to you in private, to review your history, and to assist you directly with your personal problems. Others are joined by one or more faculty members who hold group sessions. Such help can be very valuable, but as is true of other counseling activities, advisers tend to be as good or as bad as the individual chance brings your way. Experience has shown that some 20 percent find their advisers compatible and helpful. Many students either do not need—or do not acknowledge their need for—help. For such students, advisers are unlikely to be useful.

Recently students have discovered an alternative way of dealing with their difficulties at school. "Support groups" have emerged, in which students meet informally, either by themselves or together with selected advisers. Successful support groups give students the opportunity to develop new friends and allow them to share their concerns openly. Generally those who have participated find support groups quite helpful.

Students particularly vulnerable to nonacademic pressures are minorities, women, married, and older students. Representation from these groups has steadily increased over the last decade. In general, most schools have welcomed them, recognizing that diversity is far better than homogeneity. Still, isolated incidences of misunderstandings, and even outright prejudice, burden students struggling to cope with the medical school curriculum and patient care. Support groups, advisers, university health-service personnel, and in some schools, chaplains, are available to help. Seek their aid if you feel it might help you. Do not permit yourself to be ensnarled in a mesh of emotional turmoil because of your particular circumstances.

All Work and No Play?

Surprisingly, despite the heavy workload, anxiety about absorbing mountains of material, and participation in the overachieving, competitive medical-school environment, students discover that they still have time to spend on their personal lives and on extracurricular activities. Opportunities do exist for nonscheduled, nonrequired scholarly pursuits, especially at some large universities where, as an added benefit, medical students may take college and graduate courses elsewhere on campus without charge.

Students also become involved in student government, school committees, and national organizations. Some even serve on curriculum and admissions committees and occasionally even on search committees to find new faculty. At certain schools students have organized special courses and have been asked to evaluate the curriculum.

Since medical schools are frequently located on the same campus as the university's college and graduate departments, social activities tend to be similar to events that were open to you as an undergraduate: films, lectures, dances, and the like. At a number of medical schools students can participate in theatrical performances usually created as a satire of faculty, fellow students, and the medical profession in general.

4.
Your
First
Steps

While You're Still in High School

It is not too early to plan for medical school while you're in high school. Most students take the traditional route; that is, after graduating from high school they go to a four-year college, and then, in their senior year, apply to medical school. Even so, many students, who already consider a medical career seriously, wonder about which college they should go to and which major they should choose. Many think that it might be best to go to a smaller, perhaps less prestigious school, where they might have a chance at standing out. Or would it be better to go to a highly acclaimed institution and emerge as a solid but mid-level student? There is no way of telling. The admission process is so open to chance that it's impossible to know how your admissions committee will react to your record.

In the long run, and for your own well-being, it's probably best to choose a college you like. If it's the prime reason for going, you're even likely to do your best there academically, anyway. Your college represents four very important years. Many people look back over their undergraduate days and feel that they were the most important in their lives. It would be tragic if you were to waste those years as merely stepping-stones to medical school.

If you choose a college principally because it may be the best route to medical school, it could easily backfire. Your unhappiness there could cause you to lack motivation, undermining your undergraduate academic success. Or letters of recommendation from your college professors may subtly reveal that you were a maladjusted student there.

Following the same reasoning, the choice of your major should be dictated primarily by your interest in the subject, not by a too careful analysis about how it will get you into medical school. While science majors have traditionally dominated the freshman class at most medical schools, it is no longer so certain that there is an overwhelming advantage to selecting a particular college major. Admissions committees today look upon excellence in whatever major you choose as the prime criterion for selection. Choose the major and the college that will allow you to enjoy your undergraduate years. Your enthusiasm is quite likely to translate into academic success and, helpfully, good letters of recommendation. (See "Your College Major," page 90.)

Of course, you should choose a college that offers a

sufficient number of science and other courses that will be required by most medical schools. (See the directory at the back of the book for medical school undergraduate course requirements.) And you should certainly apply to schools with high standards and quality faculty, whether they are among the most prestigious or little-known colleges.

One thing that might be good is for you to discover whether the college you select has had a good track record in sending graduates to medical school. It also might be wise to learn if there is a pre-med advisory staff on campus and how competent they are. You'll do well to get this information from currently enrolled students on campus who are interested in a medical career. They'll know about the kind of support offered and where the school's graduates have been admitted.

College Level Examination Program

Some high school students may earn college credit for studies performed outside of the classroom. The College Level Examination Program (CLEP) offers tests in thirty subject areas, plus five general exams in liberal arts. Your college determines whether or not to accept credit earned this way. For details, write to

CLEP
Educational Testing Service
P.O. Box 1822
Princeton, NJ 08541.

Approximately 75 percent of U.S. medical schools have accepted CLEP credits, so long as your undergraduate school permitted them.

Combined Undergraduate/Medical School Programs

Today, eleven U.S. schools offer, on a single university campus, a combined baccalaureate/medical school program, leading to an M.D. degree. Some of these programs are limited to state residents. The most difficult part about deciding whether these programs are for you is the challenge of making such a momentous decision at such an early stage in your life. Perhaps, if you read this book and think seriously about the medical profession, its changing styles, its demands and expectations, its emotional and intellectual challenges, you may be in a better position to assess whether you are ready to commit yourself to a medical career now.

Clearly these programs have been successful. Graduates have gone on to do well in medicine. As a matter of fact, it is the traditional way for students to earn their medical degrees in Europe. In the U.S., students who enter these programs agree overwhelmingly that they made their commitment to medicine early and that all of their subsequent academic activities were centered on that goal. If you are like them, consider these programs seriously. They can be quite attractive, offering you the tremendous advantage of removing your anxiety about getting into medical school later on. Another major benefit is that such programs allow students to take courses that excite them, broadening their academic experience, without the worry over whether each course contributes to their portfolio for medical school.

Admittance to these B.A. or B.S./M.D. programs is based on your high-school record. Once admitted, you should expect it to take six or seven years to complete your M.D. degree. If you are interested, write to the schools that offer these plans. Those that currently offer the medical school and undergraduate division on one campus are:

Boston University
Brown
Case Western Reserve
Louisiana State, Shreveport (state residents only)
Miami
University of Michigan
University of Missouri, Kansas City
Northwestern
Ohio, Northeastern (state residents only)
Washington University, St. Louis
University of Wisconsin (state residents only)

Medical schools that currently offer these programs with other undergraduate institutions are:

University of California, Los Angeles (UCLA)
Hahnemann
Jefferson
University of Maryland (state residents only)
SUNY, Albany
SUNY, Downstate (state residents only)

Medical College of Pennsylvania
Ponce
Medical College of Wisconsin

Addresses are listed in the directory at the back of this book.

5.
Applying
To
Medical
School

Before tackling the details of applying and actually filling out your applications to medical schools, keep in mind that two key aspects of the application process play a central role in influencing the likelihood of your being accepted. The first and most important is *your academic profile,* including your grade-point average, college major, MCAT scores, letters of recommendation, extracurricular activities, and—at almost all schools—your interview.

Not universally appreciated but very significant is the second principal feature in the application process—*luck*. If your academic record is remarkably strong or, conversely, easily identified as very weak, luck plays a much less critical role. But for the large number of applicants who fall between these two extremes, luck figures prominently. Luck is especially important for the well-qualified applicant: the student who is neither outstandingly brilliant nor below acceptable standard; the student with good grades, decent MCAT scores, and fine letters of recommendation.

It is fair to say that most admissions committee members would be offended by the use of the word *luck*. Instead they might suggest that acceptance or rejection is based on differing value judgments or on the interests of different members of the admissions committee. What's more, if there was a chance that "luck" could possibly imply unfair treatment, they would be correct in maintaining that each application is given a fair and appropriate appraisal.

All schools insist that no single factor in an applicant's record predominates or emerges as the deciding factor in the selection process. They claim that each applicant's entire academic record is given a fair, overall evaluation. Yet it would be foolish to ignore the fact that certain minimal standards are demanded and that failure to meet them can place you out of the running from the start.

Published data on the academic profiles of students admitted to medical schools in the United States reveal a pattern of those most likely to gain acceptance. To better appreciate your chances it would be good to review information available from those schools you may be considering. At the back of this book you'll find a summary of important data available from all schools in the U.S. and Canada. Each spring the American Association of Medical Colleges issues a comprehensive paperback guide, *Medical School Admission Requirements*. It would be wise for you to get a copy.

Screening Your Application

The first step in moving your application along is the initial screening. Schools have various methods and committees to decide on the initial application. Some schools enlist the aid of one or more members of their admissions committee. Others empower a separate screening committee to review each application to decide if further consideration, including an interview, is appropriate.

At this early stage the number of applications presented to these screening groups exceeds the number of applicants who can reasonably be expected to be asked to come for an interview. Obviously students with exceptional academic records are almost uniformly selected for the interview, while very weak students are often targeted for rejection.

Your Grade-point Average

Your grade-point average (GPA) is a key element in your total academic record. Both your *science* GPA and your *cumulative* GPA for all courses greatly influence the admission committee's initial impression of your application.

Committee members—in a manner known only to themselves—measure the relative weight of GPAs from different schools on an imperfect balance. Most believe that a GPA earned at one school is a more significant mark of achievement than the very same GPA from, say, a "less competitive, less prestigious" college. Since no two members of any admissions committee would agree on objective criteria for these weighting judgments, it is unlikely that schools will ever publish universally accepted criteria for what they now do by subjective guesswork.

The relative impact of your GPA depends, in part, on the types of courses you had as an undergraduate. For example, a science GPA of 3.3 where the student has taken difficult courses at an advanced level is viewed differently from a higher science average without those advanced classes. Students often avoid high-level courses, lest they run the risk of blemishing their good record. Yet it is difficult to say with assurance whether such action is wise or ill-considered. Obviously, getting good grades in one or more advanced-level courses can be a distinct advantage.

Other factors can also influence the interpretation of your GPA. Some students, for example, discover that their overall GPA covering their four years of college is not as high as they would like it to be, given the competition from other students. Yet, to their great relief, they learn that admissions committees can often interpret favorably a steadily moving trend from freshman through senior year. What's more, if your GPA is significantly altered by grades received from one or two courses taken away from your primary campus, these may or may not contribute significantly to a favorable interpretation. Also, some admissions committees may raise questions about your ability to adjust to a single medical school environment if your record shows that you attended a large number of undergraduate colleges.

Advanced Placement Credits

Many medical schools accept "advanced placement credits," based on high-school performance or special placement exams. Since not all medical schools accept these credits, make sure that you list them appropriately. To avoid problems your transcript should meet the requirements of each medical school to which you apply. Consequently it is wise to write to each school long in advance, to receive their special instructions on how to apply, what elements are acceptable, and which are not.

College Course Requirements

Each school outlines what it considers to be a basic set of undergraduate required courses, prior to entering medical school. In general, however, most schools require a year of college biology, two years of chemistry, and a year of physics. Beyond these basic courses, some schools also require or recommend additional courses in mathematics and/or biochemistry. Specific requirements of each school are listed at the end of this book. The American Association of Medical Colleges updates this information each spring in its book, *Medical School Admission Requirements*. You can also get very specific data on each school's requirements by writing to the admissions department for a brochure.

Medical College Admissions Test

The Medical College Admissions Test (MCAT) is required by almost all schools. Even those that do not insist that you take it may still use the results in deciding between two otherwise comparable candidates. So it pays to get good MCAT scores. The MCAT evaluates your knowledge in biology, chemistry, and physics.

A test assessing your reading skills and problem-solving abilities has just been added. It is still too early to assess the effect that these recent changes will have on admissions committees. In April 1985, the new experimental section requiring an essay is incorporated into the MCAT and is likely to become a regular part of the examination thereafter. What effect this will have on the profile of the entering 1986 class and other classes beyond is speculative at best; but be advised that you will need to write an essay in response to a question based on a short narrative. Obviously a neat, correctly spelled, and coherently organized exposition, using good grammar and logical thinking, will be viewed with favor. But how the essay will be graded or evaluated and how each school will use it in its overall assessment of each candidate's performance is a matter of conjecture.

Because it is a standard evaluation that compares all applicants on a single scale, the MCAT is considered a very important item by admissions committees. The MCAT is not only a standard by which to compare individuals applying in a given year, but it also offers an objective method for analyzing current students with those from years past.

MCATs also help evaluate the variability in GPAs

from different schools. A high GPA at a less competitive school, accompanied by a poor MCAT score, often is not viewed with favor. Conversely a top-notch MCAT score, associated with mid-level GPAs at a relatively "tough school," can rescue an application from the rejection pile.

To gain insight into the style and content of the MCAT, consult the American Association of Medical Colleges' booklet on admission requirements and also the *MCAT Student Manual,* also available from the Association of American Medical Colleges.

The MCAT is given in the fall and spring of each year. Since the deadline for admission for most schools is November 1, plus or minus a month on either side, you are well advised to take the test no later than September of the year of application. If your application is received prior to the deadline, schools will hold your file open until the MCAT scores are reported. Students must advise MCAT examiners when and where to send their scores.

Many recommend that you take the examination in April, at the end of your junior year. This allows an early review of your completed application, considered by many to be a distinct advantage. At this point in your education you undoubtedly will have just completed your pre-med science requirements. Since science especially will be tested by the MCAT, you should be at the peak of preparation. Such a schedule also gives you a chance to retake the examination in September if you do not do well on your first try.

While MCAT scores are considered very important by most schools, they certainly do not account exclusively for admission or rejection. Surprisingly, many students with extremely high MCAT scores, plus very high GPAs, end up being rejected. What's more, other students with significantly lower scores surprise everyone and are admitted. Remember: A composite picture of your entire academic career and portfolio is reviewed carefully before a decision is rendered. A single element may not be as significant as a combination of different factors.

The MCAT does not offer a makeup exam, but if for religious reasons or because of unavoidable conflicts you cannot take the test when scheduled—usually on Saturdays in April and September each year—special Sunday exams can be arranged. In 1984, the MCAT fee was $50, plus $5 for special Sunday tests.

The MCAT packet—including a registration card and information about exam dates, locations, score distributions, and deadlines—is usually available at the end of January each year and can be obtained from your pre-med adviser or at the nearest college or university testing center. Or write to

MCAT Registration
The American College Testing Program
P.O. Box 414
Iowa City, IA 52243.

Your MCAT results will automatically be sent to all AMCAS participating schools to which you apply. In addition, your MCAT fee entitles you to have your test scores sent free of charge to six non-AMCAS schools of your choice. Two copies of your score report will also be sent directly to you. One is for your own records; the other should be sent to your pre-med adviser.

Excuses

In this environment your why-I-didn't-do-so-well letter sent along to your committee has little impact. Admissions committees are inundated with many creative reasons to explain suboptimal performance at a particular sitting for this examination. Most of these are considered amusing diversions during the arduous, and not infrequently boring, process of reviewing hundreds of applications. Explanations for inadequate performance usually fall into two categories: illness and distraction.

Each committee member reacts to a claim of illness on an individual basis, but usually members are not persuaded. The chance of illness reinforces the advantage of taking the MCAT in April, giving you another opportunity in September.

Distractions offer an even less viable excuse. Such horrendous events as an applicant going into premature labor in the next seat, band practice outside the window, a teeth-grinding participant seated directly behind you, and the like evoke more amusement than sympathy. These excuses can turn into committee lunchroom amusement, but they do not generate a letter of acceptance. On balance, such letters probably have a negative effect.

Letters of Recommendation

A good letter of recommendation is an important and invaluable asset in your quest for admission. At many colleges pre-medical advisory committees, which counsel students, also generate letters of recommendation. The letter from your undergraduate advisory group is usually a composite of other letters prepared by the college faculty, usually at your request.

Alternatively, you may ask faculty members individually to send letters of recommendation to the schools you've selected. Most medical schools limit the number of these letters and also suggest that a share of them come from your college faculty, preferably those in science departments.

Selecting authors for these letters is very important and should be undertaken with great care. Do not assume that the most flattering letter will come from the professor who gave you the best grade. A good grade, obtained mainly from your skills at performing well on an examination, may not translate into a noteworthy letter of recommendation. Many medical schools in their instructions to letter-authors ask for comments on a wide variety of your scholarly and general characteristics—your integrity, motivation, honesty, congeniality, work ethic, and ability to understand basic concepts and to solve problems, among other issues.

Before you choose authors for such significant letters, ask yourself, "Do they like me? Do they know me well enough to comment on my attributes, other than my academic standing? Did we get along?" You might also ask yourself if your letter-writers are aware of your other activities on and off campus.

Once you've decided who it would be best to approach, your request should be made under circumstances that allow a few minutes for discussion. A chance meeting in the hall or the parking lot is not an opportune moment. Also try to judge how enthusiastic the proposed letters are likely to be. Rather than asking, perhaps too simply, "Will you write a letter for me?" you might ask if they feel they are in a position to support your application. And you might also tell them things about yourself and your academic life that might assist them in writing about you. In discussing your career and your hopes for the future, you may even convey your genuine commitment to medicine and the importance of letters of recommendation in your quest. Ultimately your letter-writers may be delighted and eager to provide you with vigorous support.

Of course, you may come upon those who appear reluctant and hesitant. It's best to extricate yourself quickly from such a situation and to seek recommendations from others.

When you approach your letter-writers, make certain that they understand what medical schools want to know about you: how well you accept responsibility; how thorough you are in completing assigned tasks; and how well you perform in the lab. The letters should answer these questions: Do you express yourself well? Are you good at concept formation and problem solving? Are you pleasant and easy to work with? The letter-writers ought to state whether their evaluation is based on a relationship that emerged through a classroom experience or at certain extracurricular activities. It is highly recommended that you give your letter-writers a one-page resume, outlining your activities, to help them with details. Encourage them to insert a personal note expressing their views about you. It would also be good to have one or two specific examples about your work or your life that make you an attractive candidate.

How many letters should you submit? Submit the

numbers asked for in each school's application form. If you must, exceed that limit by one at most. During the active admission period, committee members are overloaded with work. Extra letters mean extra work and extra time. The arrival of additional letters also raises questions about your sense of security. Why so many letters? Committee members begin to wonder whether you are confident in your expectations of receiving a good recommendation. You may have asked for many more than necessary to be sure of at least one or two good ones. Good judgment— your ability to know how you did and to be confident about it—is an important trait. Excessive numbers of letters raise questions about your ability to judge how other people perceive your worth.

Who should write your letter? Your strongest support will come from those faculty members who know you more than merely as a student in their classroom. They know you because you have become involved with them in some working relationship, say, in one of your research projects. Or you may have worked closely with them on a school committee or in any of a number of ways, outside of large classroom settings.

Other than college faculty, physicians with whom you have worked can also write useful letters. But avoid relying on physicians who are friends or relatives. As it becomes clear that your relationship with the doctor was more familial than collegial, the letter becomes vanishingly important. The committee is looking for as many objective assessments of your qualifications as they can review. A family booster is likely to backfire.

Recommendations that arrive late rarely influence decisions about your application. The sudden discovery by a newfound benefactor at the eleventh hour who claims that you are greater than anyone who had ever applied to medical school raises more doubts about your judgment and none about the committee's.

Extracurricular Activities

Perhaps the most misunderstood contribution to your portfolio is your extracurricular activities. Myths about the power and the pursuit of extracurricular work mislead many students into taking summer jobs as bedpan orderlies, ward assistants, and marauders in emergency rooms of general hospitals.

Obviously medical schools are looking for students who have done more than acquire good grades and good rankings. While it is true that for many years it was recommended that students restrict their nonacademic pursuits to health care, today, after a long period of gradual change, the best-qualified candidate is not someone who has succeeded in securing a dead-end ward job but one who has demonstrated abilities over a wide variety of activities. For example, you may now show your interpersonal skills as a teacher or counselor, or your creative abilities as a program director, developing an innovative new plan. Your scholastic depth can be demonstrated by writing a book, a major piece of research, or a computer program. And your knowledge and concern with important social issues might emerge from your assignment as a legislative aide. Any activity that permits you to emerge as an individual with a broad cultural background would demonstrate your maturity and sense of purpose. On campus all sorts of activities not only show your human qualities but also are wise choices for your medical career. These range from campus politics to team sports. Your music, art, dance, and other creative talents are also happy inclusions in your portfolio.

Medical school committees have acknowledged that achievement in your extracurricular activities can indicate your ability to define goals, make commitments, persevere, and ultimately succeed. These attributes can be shown in many areas and need not be revealed exclusively in health care. If you are lucky enough to accomplish these goals within a health-care environment, your committee will surely look favorably upon your efforts. So, by all means pursue a creative, demanding role in a hospital or other health-care setting. But don't feel that because you helped carry bedpans one summer you demonstrated your special creative talents and interpersonal skills. If that was its aim, your summer may have been entirely wasted.

Sad, but true, for most students, the impact of their extracurricular activities, more than any other aspect of their credentials, is susceptible to luck. Remember that your completed application is presented to an individual or to a group who perform first-line screening. Your MCAT scores and GPAs are less likely to invoke subjective responses. When the admissions committee turns to your extracurricular activities, however, objective evaluations are less obvious. Your committee cannot avoid viewing your after-school life, your social involvements, and your human qualities against a background of their own value systems. They will interpret your nonacademic performance, choice, and style in the light of their own interests and goals.

Of course, accomplishment as a classical pianist is viewed much more favorably when, just by chance, a key committee member reviewing your record is an amateur classical musician. Your athletic prowess will be viewed variously by members of the committee, depending, naturally, on their attitude toward the role of sports in a scholastic environment. One medical school professor on the committee may be thrilled by a student's portfolio containing innovative and creative computer programming capabilities, while another member is unnerved by computers. And a psychiatrist on your committee may be remarkably interested in the student who worked at a halfway house, helping to rehabilitate psychologically disturbed children.

It is worth repeating: No one will match your application with just the perfect screening committee member who fully appreciates your interests and concerns. Chances are just as good that your folder will end up in the least sympathetic hands, as in the hands of your champion. It is totally random—or just plain luck.

If you have engaged in a scientific research project in college, medical school committees usually see that as an asset. And it should come as no surprise. Most medical school faculty members are appointed to their positions mostly on the basis of their research. They are very committed to their work and have devoted their life's work to science. They feel that an understanding of the basic concepts of scientific inquiry and scientific method is an essential part of being a good physician, even if you do not undertake a lifetime career in research. Since most faculty members on admissions committees hold research experience as a valuable contribution to your medical education, they will allow their views to appropriately influence their evaluation of your credentials along these lines.

Your College Major

History shows that, until today, most medical schools favored, if they did not require, a science major as a prerequisite for admission.

Yet a slow, quiet, and as-yet unquestioned change is taking place. Schools are accepting an increasing percentage of nonscience majors. On today's medical school campuses music, art, and literature majors are numerous and are even considered a valuable asset to the scholarly community. What's more, nonscience majors have demonstrated their ability to do well in the rigorous medical school program. The change is due, in part, as a response to years of criticism in which medical schools have been accused of a selection process that relied almost exclusively on science majors and high test scores.

But be warned: If you are a nonscience major, luck may play a decisive role in whether you are admitted. Those reviewing your application may be totally unimpressed with your accomplishments in eighteenth-century poetry or atonal music. Still, your chances have improved significantly from years ago. Consider these rather striking statistics: Of the 1983–84 entering class, approximately 40 percent were biological science undergraduate majors. Another 20 percent had majored in the physical sciences. The remaining 40 percent came from nonscience or other disciplines.

Your Application

Approximately 100 medical schools participate in the American Medical College Application Service (AMCAS). Under this plan all you need do is complete a single application. It is then sent on to the participating schools you seek to enter. Nonparticipating schools require that you complete separate applications.

At the back of this handbook, where each school's data is given, you'll note that under the heading, "Application and Acceptance," some schools indicate an AMCAS filing date. This notation indicates that the school is one of those participating in the American Medical College Application Service. If you are a transfer student or are seeking advanced standing, you must apply directly to the schools of your choice, even if they are among participating AMCAS institutions. Once your AMCAS application has been processed, each individual school will notify you about any further requirements.

Students pay a $30 fee, if they wish to apply to only one AMCAS-participating school. An extra $13 is charged for each additional application. Later on, some AMCAS schools will add another fee for candidates who look promising. The AMCAS may waive fees when payment may stand in the way of applying. For nonparticipating AMCAS schools, application fees range up to $60 and may be requested at different times in the application process. Fee waivers can be obtained if you provide supportive evidence from your financial-aid office. Fees for the current year are given at the back of this book under each school's listing. To obtain AMCAS application forms and other materials, submit an Application Request Form, usually available from your pre-med adviser, or write to

AMCAS
Division of Student Services
Association of American Medical Colleges
Suite 301
1776 Massachusetts Avenue, N.W.
Washington, D.C. 20036-1989
(202) 828-0600.

In addition to seeking standard biographical data, all applications ask you to indicate the sources of your letters of recommendation. For many a brief essay is also required. What's more, you will be asked to complete a number of ancillary documents—labels for returning status request cards, addresses for verifying letters of recommendation, and so on.

It is important to complete all of the required documents neatly and accurately. It's a good idea to type them. An incomplete, inaccurate, or sloppy application can impress your screening committee with your disinterest, low level of enthusiasm, and inability to accept responsibility. All of which will contribute to having your application viewed with suspicion.

Your written essay gives you a unique opportunity to present yourself as a desirable candidate. Conversely, it can also reveal that you are not worthy of serious consideration. The choice is yours. Based on my experience, I'd say that your essay is seen in the best light when it is brief, neat, and contains grammatically correct sentences with properly spelled words. Most committees look upon the essay as a chance to have students demonstrate their ability to put together a coherent piece of writing.

It's best to submit your application long in advance of deadlines set by the schools you select. At the back of this book you'll find a list of all medical schools in the U.S. and Canada. Along with other pertinent data, each school lists application filing and other deadlines. To be safe you should apply at least ten months in advance of your college graduation date.

When you apply to schools participating in the American Medical College Application Service (AMCAS), the filing deadline is the last day your AMCAS application will be accepted. For other schools the deadline is the last date you may submit your initial application form; you will be notified later if additional items are requested: transcripts, letters of recommendation, and other details. Also note that schools publish separate deadlines for their Early Decision Plans.

Your Interview

Once your committee has performed the initial screening of your application, you will be notified of the results. At best you will be asked to come in for an interview. At worst you will be rejected. Or you may be notified that you have been placed on a waiting list. The offer of an interview or the receipt of a rejection letter is a very clear-cut response to your application. But the "hold" category can be ambiguous.

If you are offered an interview, many schools will also give you the option of being seen on campus or, alternatively, in your region (either by a resident alumnus on your college campus or by a visiting admissions committee team). Many disagree over whether a regional interview carries the same weight as one on the medical school campus. But, in my view, because of the value of visiting the medical school for its own sake, the dispute over regional versus on-campus interviews fades away.

Often schools will be generous in setting your interview date to help fit it into your circuit, if you are also traveling to other schools. Requests for interviews from applicants who "just happen to be in the neighborhood" and who have not been invited are generally not granted. What's more, these requests are seen as inappropriate attempts to bypass the usual selection process.

Once you survive the screening process, your interview emerges as the most important determinant of your chances of being offered a position in the next freshman class. Now your letters of recommendation, which played an important part in the initial screening, are elevated to an even greater importance. No doubt, your interviewer will critically review them before reaching a final decision.

Here, again, luck enters the scene. And, very likely, it plays its biggest role. By its very nature the interview is a highly subjective event. A "good impression" depends on many facets of what you bring to the drama: your appearance, your self-confidence, your ability to speak well, among other attributes. But, as with any chance encounter between two strangers, your interview may happily evolve into a warm, comfortable, mutually enjoyable interchange or, sadly, turn into an awkward, cold, devastating experience. At that particular hour on that particular day you and your interviewer are each subject to different intellectual and psychological challenges, different levels of anxiety, different feelings of comfort. Sometimes there is what has been called "chemistry," which makes two people click together. At other times it just doesn't work, no matter how hard you try. The elusive "chemistry" between people may explain why two interviewers—evaluating the same applicant, hours or even minutes apart—can come away with totally different impressions. How well the two participants mesh is indeed luck—totally unpredictable and often inexplicable. Common interests, background, life-style, personal experiences, etc., all play a role. While interview assignments are mostly made at random, there is a chance that—if you are a woman or a minority candidate—you may be seen by an appropriate interviewer.

It is difficult to prepare for your interview. One person might ask the common question, "Why do you want to be a doctor?" And while you might be fully prepared to respond to it, you might easily be thrown by a surprising question. Another interviewer might ask instead, "Why didn't you choose law?" Of course, as a general rule, your interviewer will be responsive to your ability to answer questions in a concise, well-organized, and articulate manner. Try not to ramble. Answer the question and then stop. It's good to be prepared to ask about the school, the curriculum, the town. What the school has to offer that will entice you is as important as what you have to offer as a prospective student and alumnus.

It's best to appear confident but not pompous; eager to gain admission but not panic-stricken. Be neat, but try to be comfortable. Try not to be among those who engender such comments as, "He must have worn a rented suit" or "She would have been more comfortable wearing jeans."

Probably the most important aspect of your interview is your ability to talk about yourself and your interests in a way that makes your academic and other interests seem revealing and rewarding. It's good to talk about your experiences from different angles: what you accomplished, what you learned, what effect you had on others.

You should also be prepared to talk about your undergraduate research project, what was done, and, most revealing, why it was done. You should be able to speak about it in the context of the larger scientific issues in which it fits and especially how your research illuminated some aspect of a modern scientific puzzle. Your responses will reveal whether you profoundly appreciate the scientific questions or whether your participation was merely at the level of a technician.

Most likely you will be asked to come to two separate interviews, each lasting thirty to forty-five minutes. Some schools, however, will only seek one interview with you. At other schools your interviewer will be joined by medical students who are also members of admissions committees. More often a medical student will serve as your tour guide and provide you with resource services. Most schools arrange gatherings where applicants and students already enrolled are given a chance to meet and talk. These sessions offer potential newcomers the opportunity to assess the attitudes and opinions of those who have already been accepted and are now in medical school.

When facilities are available, some schools encourage applicants to arrive the day before the interview and to stay with a student on campus. If you are given the chance, take it. It is your best way of getting to know other students, and it gives you special insights into campus social life and how the school functions in its town or city. What's more, you might even be given the chance to sit in on a class or two.

Be warned: Your parents should *not* go to your interviews with you. It does not speak well of your maturity or your independence. If your parents must accompany you, have them wait in the car, at the train station, or in the airport, but don't let it be known that they are around. They must never participate.

And a special plea to parents: Leave your children alone. Don't make sure that your child has asked all the right questions, received all the proper brochures, and completed all the proper forms. The situation is anxiety-ridden enough, without adding to it.

And one final note to applicants on their way to an interview: Don't be rude to anyone. Of course, this is a general rule of conduct you ought to follow, anyway; but under heightened, anxiety-prone conditions, inadvertently you may be discourteous to seemingly "unimportant" people at the medical school: security guards, receptionists, secretaries, and others. Don't. These people may be colleagues and friends of people who are sitting on your committee or at your interview. Their negative impressions can be made known to medical school faculty and administrators.

Don't try to force an early assessment of your chances. You are expected to know that competition is fierce and that decisions cannot be made until all applicants are seen and evaluated. Even if they were inclined to do so, members of your committee cannot independently determine your fate. The selection is a communal decision.

While many students write a note to each interviewer, thanking them, expressing interest in the school, and reaffirming their commitment to medicine, it does them no great harm, but it usually is of little value. Excessive assertions about how important it is that you be at this particular school can be irritating, since the interviewer must assume that you've sent similar pleas to other schools; therefore, your ardor is discounted.

Still, good, solid reasons for your high preference for the school, stated clearly and soundly, might be helpful, since it is not a common approach. For example, your wife or husband already lives in the area. Or you might have a pressing need to be near your family. Such justified and verifiable reasons might influence your committee.

When Will You Know?

What now? It's all over and in the hands of fate. What will happen? When will you know? How did you do? What are your chances? Certainly all good questions; unfortunately, you'll not know the answers until time allows the process slowly to unfold.

Great diversity exists among schools—how and under what schedule they inform applicants. Some, with "rolling" admission policies, let you know within a week or so. They'll inform you quickly whether you've been accepted, rejected, or put on a waiting list. Others hold a big selection meeting, only two or three times a year during the November to March application cycle. These schools let you know their decisions later, once their meeting comes to an end. Neither calling nor writing will enhance your chances or speed the process.

Waiting Lists

Most frustrating is learning that you've been placed on "hold." What does it mean? Generally it means that your application is not strong enough to command immediate early acceptance, and, fortunately, not out of the running. Happily, a significant number of students on waiting lists ultimately are accepted each year. Since the first offers go to the very best students, who are frequently accepted at many schools, places open up for others, as top students select the *one* school for them. As they withdraw they are replaced by others who have been held on waiting lists. If you've been put on hold, some schools will inform you—based on their experiences over several years—what your chances are. Others will not.

In frustration you may be on a hold list up to the day of matriculation. Such delays are sometimes caused by those students who continue to keep open more than one acceptance until the eleventh hour. The practice not only causes frustration and anxiety for other students, but these indecisive students are also resented at their future schools. Through the Association of American Medical Colleges medical schools are aware of all offers. When it is apparent that students hold more than one place, they are asked to make a final choice promptly. Those who fail to decide quickly are likely to generate ill feelings—at the school they finally decline, as well as at the one ultimately selected.

Pre-med Advisers

In general, it pays to get help from your health-profession or pre-med adviser at your college. Many are members of the National Association of Health Professional Advisers, a dedicated, well-informed group. Your adviser may be among those who are up-to-date about the admission process, the differences among schools, and your chances of getting in. They may have met with members of admissions committees and deans of admissions. Often advisers have a sense of what various schools are looking for.

Some medical schools will ask you to indicate the name of the adviser at your college responsible for your application. It's best to keep your pre-med adviser up-to-date about the status of your activities, including the schools you apply to, MCAT scores, and other details. Your adviser may help you speed along the process and may guide you in other valuable ways. Advisers are also likely to have stacks of applications, instruction guides, and other information sources on hand.

Assessing Your Chances

When assessing your chances, place yourself as a member of an imaginary admissions committee. Review your own application. How would you react to the information being presented? It's amazing how many of your own questions are answered by this simple, revealing technique.

It also helps to do some research. Each year, profiles of applicant pools, indicating who has been admitted or rejected, are published for the entire country, as well as for most individual schools. These data are available from the Association of American Medical Colleges. Remember, however, that such statistics offer generalizations. Wide variations take place within each medical school, and impressive ranges exist for MCAT scores, GPAs, and other significant elements.

Early Decision Plans

Many schools offer well-qualified students the opportunity to apply for admission under an Early Decision Plan (EDP). Students who take advantage of this approach agree to submit a single application to the school of their choice with the explicit understanding that if accepted, they will attend. If you are not accepted under these programs, your application automatically reverts to the regular pool, and you are free to apply elsewhere as you wish. Early decision applications are received and reviewed early in the year, usually by October 1, allowing for additional applications later, if you are unsuccessful.

For the exceptionally qualified student who is likely to be accepted, EDPs save a lot of time, money, and worry. Lost, however, is the opportunity to visit and compare other schools before committing yourself to only one. If you feel there are great advantages to attending one particular school, there is no doubt that the Early Decision Plan is best.

Some state-supported schools accept out-of-state applicants only if they apply through Early Decision Plans.

Other schools accept EDP students from their home state only. AMCAS-participating schools have special instructions for EDP applications. Consult the AMCAS instruction booklet for details. In the school listings in the back of this handbook you'll discover which ones offer Early Decision Plans and under what conditions.

Joint-degree Programs

When you first apply to medical school, some schools give you the chance also to apply for joint-degree programs. The most common is the combined M.D./Ph.D., offered to those students primarily interested in academic careers. Because medical school courses in basic science and graduate studies in biology often cover much the same ground, students can save a good deal of time if the medical school and the graduate program at the same, or nearby, institutions permit cross-accreditation. With luck students can acquire both degrees in six years; but seven is more usual and, rarely, it can take as long as eight years.

Similarly, many schools offer degree programs jointly with public-health schools. When cross-accreditation is permitted, students can earn an M.D./M.P.H. in as little as five years. Joint degrees are also available in other fields, but they do not tend to save the student time, since the law school curriculum, for example, is not similar to the one offered in medical school. Nonetheless, students do pursue joint degrees in law, economics, political science, urban planning, and the like.

The M.D./Ph.D. Program

Many medical schools offer a combined six- to seven-year program, leading to an M.D., plus a Ph.D., usually in the biological sciences. Those interested in a career in research or a future faculty position at a medical school should consider this opportunity. It is a long and arduous challenge, but many view it as the spawning ground of the next generation of academic scientists.

The traditional route to a faculty post at a medical school includes specialty training after medical school, followed by one or two years as a postdoctoral fellow, doing research and advanced clinical work in a specialty area. But recent advances in basic biology, coupled with increased sophistication in laboratory techniques in research, has propelled the development of these combined M.D./Ph.D. programs. Those who pursue the joint degree are often better prepared for the demanding role as a medical research scientist.

One can apply directly for initial acceptance into both programs or, alternately, one may apply to the Ph.D. program at the university's graduate biology school after completing one to two years of medical school. While this latter route is becoming quite popular and is often recommended by faculty members, it is not the only way.

When you apply, you may be seen by a joint M.D. /Ph.D. review committee or perhaps by two separate committees—one from the medical school and another from the graduate school. You may be accepted into either (or both), with the privilege of accepting one or both.

Those applicants who have already earned their Ph.D.s and then wish to undertake medical studies are not universally welcomed because some of these students have not fared well at medical school. The experiences with earlier candidates at each school often determine how your application will be received. Luck, again, will play a significant role.

Similarly, M.D./Ph.D. joint-degree graduates are not received with open arms at some graduate clinical training programs. This may be because the number of students who emerged earlier from these programs have not performed well in clinical settings. While some have done exceptionally well, a good number of others failed to live up to expectations, raising doubts about their desire to acquire clinical competence.

Medical Scientist Training Program

Some M.D./Ph.D. programs are funded by grants sponsored by the National Institutes of Health and can offer significant financial benefits to you, if you are accepted. Under these grants students receive tuition and stipends for at least six and sometimes for seven years. Considering the expense of a medical education, these plans—under the Medical Scientist Training Program (MSTP)—certainly can be attractive.

In 1983, approximately 675 students were supported by these grants. About 120 new slots open up each year. Should you apply, remember that schools are looking for top scholars who have also shown keen interest in and evidence of quality research. You may apply as an MSTP candidate after completing your undergraduate degree or during the first two years of medical school or graduate training. To qualify you must be a citizen or a permanent U.S. resident.

Since these grants provide students with annual stipends of $5,000 plus tuition, your chances of being selected are small, unless you are a first-ranking student. To learn which schools offer these programs, write to

Medical Science Training Program
Room 957
Westwood Building
National Institutes of Health
Bethesda, MD 20205
(301) 496-7981.

Other Joint Degrees

Some medical schools also offer opportunities to acquire other combined degrees—master's degrees in public health and law, and theology degrees, among others. Usually they are tailored to individual needs, so if you are interested, you should inquire at the schools you've selected to find out your options.

"Where Should I Apply?"

Undoubtedly, as you ponder the question "Where should I apply?" two parallel thoughts occupy your mind. The first, "Which school might accept me?" is closely followed by, "Which one is best for me?" Obviously the second emerges as a happy dilemma, only if you are fortunate enough to be accepted by more than one school.

First, let us consider how you might go about deciding which schools are among those you should apply to. The overriding challenge is to arrive at the best fit between your academic credentials and those schools most likely to be impressed with them. Medical schools enjoy varying degrees of prestige and, as a direct consequence, are more or less competitive, even though there is no generally agreed upon rank order among them.

In trying to assess which schools on this mythical prestige ladder fit your particular background, it's best to consult published information revealing the intellectual achievements of students who have been accepted to medical schools over the past few years. The Association of American Medical Colleges and the *Journal of the American Medical Association* publish annual profiles giving mean GPAs and MCAT scores for the most recent entering freshman class. In the back of this book you'll find similar data for all U.S. and Canadian schools.

When you study the figures, it is important to know that the numbers published fail to reveal how wide the spread is. You will not know, from a simple inspection, the lowest score each school accepts; nor will you know the highest. You will not be able to determine which schools have the widest spreads and which the narrowest. What's more, no one really knows.

While your pre-med adviser appreciates how well other students at your college may have fared in years past and may have gained valuable information from colleagues about other students at other colleges, the only wise conclusion is the obvious one: The better your record, the better your chances at the more competitive schools. Nevertheless, it is also true that some of the most prestigious schools are more willing to take chances on candidates believed to possess great potential, even without high GPAs and top MCAT scores.

How Many Schools Should You Apply To?

While you should apply to schools that as a matter of past record have accepted students with academic credentials similar to yours, because of uncertainty in your own assessment of your record, as well as in the admission process itself, you should apply to some schools with average statistics higher than yours plus a few below. Since most applicants apply to about ten schools, you should also select ten that appear to match your record. It then might not be a bad idea to add a couple above and a couple below. Then spin the wheel.

In-state vs. Out-of-state Schools

By all means apply to your state school and then to private schools. Be advised, however, that even private schools, because of state funding and capitation grants, frequently take a fixed percentage of home-state applicants. Again, consult appropriate tables in the *Journal of the American Medical Association* supplement or leaf through the statistics for each school at the back of this handbook. You'll learn how many students each school usually accepts from out of the state and how many each one accepts from its home state.

Of course, when considering the schools that might be right for you, you must consider costs and financial aid (see "Your Finances," p. 145). These considerations are especially important in weighing choices between private schools and a state-supported school in your home state.

State-supported schools are usually required by law to offer preference to their in-state applicants. Some public medical schools allow nonresidents to apply but only if admitted through Early Decision Plans. Others even have quotas by county or region within their state. Remember that tuition for in-state students is often considerably less than for nonresidents.

Obviously, because of the significant bias toward in-state applicants, your chances for admission—whether in a state-supported or a private school—are best in your home state. It is highly unlikely that you will be accepted to a public medical school in a state where you are not a resident, unless you are a top candidate.

Interstate Agreements

If your home state does not have a medical school of its own, you may discover that neighboring states may offer you certain preferences. Regional and other agreements may provide you with special opportunities. Consider the following plans.

Western Interstate Commission for Higher Education Professional Student Exchange Program. Students from

Alaska, Montana, and Wyoming are eligible. For information about how to apply, which schools accept students from this program, how much money your home state may have available for your support, and other details, write to Professional Student Exchange Program, Western Interstate Commission for Higher Education. P.O. Drawer P, Boulder, CO 80302.

The Washington, Alaska, Montana, and Idaho Program. Students from these states may be admitted to the University of Washington School of Medicine and pay tuition and fees as if they were residents of the State of Washington. For details about who is eligible and how to apply, write to WAMI Program, University of Washington SM-22, School of Medicine, Seattle, WA 98195.

New England Board of Higher Education Regional Medical Student Contract Program. If you are a resident of Massachusetts and are admitted to Boston University or Tufts University medical schools, under this program you are entitled to a reduction in your tuition in exchange for agreeing to perform, after you graduate, medical service in the state. For details contact Office of Contract Services, New England Board of Higher Education, 9 School Street, Wenham, MA 01984.

Southern Regional Education Board Program. Under this plan certain students who apply from Alabama, Florida, Georgia, Maryland, Mississippi, North Carolina, Tennessee, and Virginia and who are accepted at Meharry Medical College (in Tennessee) pay reduced tuition. Other students from Alabama who are accepted for the first two years at Morehouse School of Medicine (in Georgia) receive similar benefits. Write to Southern Regional Education Board, 1340 Spring Street N.W., Atlanta, GA 30309.

Medical School Programs

Forgetting for the moment about prestige and competition, let us consider the types of medical school programs.
Of the 127 schools in the U.S., approximately 100 offer the
traditional four-year program, divided into two years of
basic science and two years of clinical apprenticeship (see
"Clinical Clerkship," page 49). The overwhelming majority of students accepted to medical schools in the U.S. are
those who have earned their baccalaureate degrees after
completing four years of undergraduate study. Rarely, and
only for students with exceptional records, do some schools
accept students after they have completed three years of
college.

Three-year and Six-year Programs

Some medical schools allow students with advanced-level
undergraduate work (or those who have earned their
Ph.D.s in the biological sciences) to finish medical school
in three years. Currently no U.S. school offers a three-year
program to all its students.

Over the last decade approximately fourteen schools
attempted three-year programs. In the end, however,
students and faculty jointly agreed that such abbreviated
courses were ill-advised, and they have been discontinued.
Three-year medical school programs were overly com-
pressed, denied students vacations, and pressured students into career choices far too early.

Still other schools offer six- and seven-year programs.

In these students are admitted directly from high school. They provide undergraduate college courses leading to a B.A., and then go on to offer an M.D. degree at the very end. Students who enroll in these combined B.A./M.D. programs (common in Europe), must commit themselves quite early to a medical career (see "Combined Undergraduate/Medical School Programs, page 70). In return, however, students accepted to such schools are spared the competitive "pre-med syndrome."

Early Admissions

Some colleges in the U.S. promise a small number of sophomores automatic admission to the medical school at the university after they earn their undergraduate degrees. Often called "2-4 programs," these early admission options allow students to study liberal arts or take other useful courses as juniors and seniors without overly intensive concentration on the sciences and without jeopardizing their chances for acceptance to medical school (because they may engage in more unusual undergraduate scholarly activities). Since the few who are accepted to early admissions programs are those who have already demonstrated remarkable academic records (and who would undoubtedly gain admission to the medical school of their choice, anyway), these programs do not tend to be very popular.

Nevertheless, early admission programs offer advantages to exceptionally bright students. If such a program exists on your campus, it may be worthwhile for you to pursue it.

Teaching Styles and Other Aspects

Teaching styles ought also to be considered when you evaluate schools that might be right for you. Do they rely primarily on lectures or do they offer small group settings with interactive teaching? Is clinical work introduced in parallel with basic science studies? Or are basic science and clinical medicine completely separated, the first two years devoted exclusively to science and the second two entirely to practice? Are courses interdisciplinary, with teams of instructors giving various aspects of the field?

Will your academic success or failure be based on your grades, class rank, and examinations? Or is a pass/fail system in place? Does the school require that you pass National Boards for graduation or for advancement into the upper-level clinical division?

It would also be helpful to know how good the clinical facilities are at the schools you select. Where will you get your clinical training? Will you be assigned to a community hospital? Such training has distinct advantages, offering students broader clinical experience. Learn, too, where students go for their clinical clerkships.

You should also be aware that some medical schools, unaffiliated with a university or separated from the main campus of affiliated universities, may not offer cultural, academic, and social advantages that appeal to many students. Keep this in mind in making your selections.

What Are Your Chances?

Let's be realistic. Until you receive two or more accep-
tances, the fine points about which schools would be best
for you remain moot questions. Until then, you should
focus your energies on the cluster of schools most likely to
review your academic record with favor. Again, because of
"luck," it is difficult to define your chances with accuracy.

Given careful and honest assessment of your record,
what are your chances? Better than most people think,
and perhaps getting better. Last year, 40,000 students
applied to medical school, and 17,000 were admitted.
Remember that these 40,000 applicants include foreign
nationals and repeat applications. If you reduce the total
by these categories, the number was approximately 32,000.
Which means that first-time applicants have a fifty-fifty
chance of getting into medical school.

It's also important to note that the total number of
new applicants to all medical schools has decreased by 5
percent. If this trend continues, your chances increase.
What's more, if you are a minority candidate, your chances
might also be slightly better. Recent active efforts to
improve minority representation has had its effect at many
schools.

Following Up

Monitor the progress of your application. If you fear that
something is missing or that you should have heard from
the school, occasional inquiries about the status of your

application are certainly prudent and acceptable. But remember to be courteous, even when a very busy staff member fails to respond to your question. Be satisfied when you are offered a postcard or a letter to be sent later in response to your telephone inquiry. Do not demand that the status of your application be clarified immediately.

You're Accepted: Which School Is for You?

For those fortunate to be offered more than one acceptance, the choice can be perplexing and agonizing. Let's consider how to assess the various arguments favoring one school over another.

Probably the most potent influence on the side of any school is its *prestige*. While there is no official ranking, there is no doubt that some schools are viewed as being better than others. Prestige is not earned because of a school's quality education alone. Certainly the national reputation of its basic science faculty and the noted achievements of its clinical departments contribute significantly to its fame.

And make no mistake about it: Glory earned in years past plays an important role. Reputation is built over time, and achievement gained in an earlier era does not disappear easily. The major, prestigious medical schools and their associated hospitals earned their reputations from historical fact. From the turn of the century until just recently, they constituted the principal centers of research and innovative clinical practice. Well funded, they attracted the best scientists and clinicians. They could afford a large, full-time faculty, providing experts in almost all areas of science and clinical medicine.

Other schools suffered with skeleton staffs and relied largely on part-time practitioners as instructors. While these physician-professors might have been excellent clinicians, they could devote only a fraction of their time to teaching and hardly any to research. Today the difference between the top schools and the less-than-quality institutions has almost disappeared. With federal funding and other aid all schools expanded their faculties, entered sophisticated research, and now compete successfully for national recognition as clinical centers. To expand their faculties many professors were recruited from the prestigious schools and, like many junior athletes, became as good as their coaches.

Still, there are advantages to being a graduate from one of the prestigious schools. It may be somewhat overrated, but it can play a part in how others interpret your credentials, not only at the time of graduation but also subsequently, when you apply for jobs.

But, as with most things, there are two sides to this question. When you apply for your postgraduate training or for a position later on, is it better to be a top student from a mid-level medical school or just an average one from a high-ranking school? Of course, postgraduate directors are eager to attract graduates from the prestigious schools. Yet they also perceive of their departments as national resources, so they seek students from other schools throughout the country. No director selects more than a few students from any one school, which leaves you wondering whether you'd rather emerge as the golden student from a modest school or an average one from one of the glamour schools.

As you look into the future there may be other advantages to being a graduate from one of the prestigious schools. In the next decades, as more physicians are employed by hospitals, industry, health-maintenance organizations, for-profit medical-care companies, and the like, your medical-school credentials will emerge as an important factor in your ability to make wide career choices.

The bottom line is that all schools now offer you the opportunity to become as good a physician as your ability and your motivation dictate. So does it matter? Let's consider the myths that may be associated with your choice.

The Career Myth. Let us suppose that you plan to be a neurosurgeon. Since School A is thought to be strong in neurosurgery, you select it as your top choice. Bad reasoning. First of all, at this early stage in your career, you cannot predict whether your commitment to neurosurgery will last. Once you are exposed to all the specialties and you gain an appreciation of the types and styles of practice in each—most of which you are not unaware—you may very well change your mind. Experience shows that most students end up choosing an area of medicine not at all like the one they first had in mind. What's more, the medical school you attend plays a minor role in your ultimate ability to gain access to a particular discipline. You'll find that your practice will depend principally on what happens *after* graduation—especially your residency and fellowship training program.

The Location Myth. Most students think that they ought to go to school in the area where they ultimately plan to practice. But, again, statistics show that most physicians end up practicing in the area of their postgraduate training rather than in the part of the country where their medical school is located. So it's best to ignore location, even if you think it matters now.

Bottom-line Advice

All other things being equal, if you have the choice, you are likely to select the more prestigious school. But while this choice is understandable, you should also keep in mind that personal, financial, or other reasons may make another school more desirable. Don't feel that you're losing out by passing up the chance to go to one of the "better" schools.

In making your choice you should consider a broad range of questions that may be more important to you than prestige: location or proximity to your home (or, alternatively, the desire to be away from home); a relationship with another student; the campus environment; and programs offered. You will have to work very hard for four years, and anything you do to ease your burden is worthy of serious consideration. Remember that among the many distinguished leaders at the forefront of medical science are graduates from practically every medical school in the country.

6.
Your
Special
Background

Older Applicants

If you are an older applicant, you may experience a somewhat more difficult time gaining admission to medical school. This won't be because of your age itself but, rather, because of questions that may be raised about an older applicant's decision to enter a medical career. Once again (as has often been repeated here), chance and coincidence will play a key role in whether you are admitted or even considered. The attitudes of admissions committee members who consider your application (and your interviewer) will be very important in deciding your fate.

You may face tough opposition by some committee members who may worry about your late decision to enter medicine. Biased or not, they will be concerned that you may be among those who are "perpetual" students, who seek admission to medical school after years of continual degree-earning. They may feel that your aim is to pursue medical studies to avoid responsibility outside of academic life. In this case your goal may not be to practice medicine but just to continue going to school.

Some older students may not have achieved the kind of success they had hoped for themselves in other walks of life—research, business, teaching, or another field. They turn to medicine as an alternative, perhaps to gain the success that eluded them elsewhere. Some who are successful in other fields may look to medicine, as cutbacks in federal support, declines in teaching programs, and other obstacles at their work make medicine attractive. Recently, for example, as support for research has declined, Ph.D. applicants to medical school have increased, raising the suspicion that these students are looking to medicine as a more generous source of funding.

Older applicants, of course, have a shorter future professional life ahead. Should the school deny a medical education to younger students with a longer potential career?

Older students must convince admissions committee members that they possess a genuine commitment to medicine. They must show that their late decision to enter medical school has been made on solid grounds. Older applicants must reveal that their earlier choices do not stand in their way but actually reinforce their understanding of the profession. Qualities and skills earned elsewhere will be useful and important. Your earlier activities— educational, professional, or in business—may be a decisive asset to your long-range career goals. For instance, a physicist with experience in the technology of CAT-scanning, nuclear magnetic resonance, or laser beams brings superior talent to the profession. As an older applicant you can make a creditable argument that your career in business or economics can be fruitfully applied to hospital administration or other significant medical fields. Your long-standing commitment to the social sciences, which would be enhanced by a medical degree, can make a quite reasonable presentation to your admissions committee.

No school has (or admits to having) a policy that discriminates against applicants on the basis of their age. What's more, over the last decade, the number of older students admitted to medical school has increased, suggesting that traditional attitudes of restricting access to those over twenty-five have changed.

Older students should keep in mind that medical school is an arduous task, requiring long hours and hard work. It may impinge significantly on a life-style to which you may have become accustomed. Family obligations compete with study and clinical commitments. As you serve your clerkship and subsequently as a house officer, a tremendous strain is placed on your family relationships. But if you are certain that medicine is for you, by all means apply.

Women

In the last ten years the number of women in medical school has risen impressively. Approximately 30 percent of all students are now women, matching a 30 percent female applicant pool. The historical policy of limiting the number of women in medical school is gone. Undoubtedly we can expect a continued rise in the number of women applicants until, one day, approximately 50 percent of the student body will be women. Furthermore, women medical school graduates no longer pursue traditional "female specialties" alone—pediatrics and psychiatry—but are now taking their rightful place in all medical disciplines, including conventionally male-dominated surgical specialties. Generally speaking, the medical profession and medical schools have adjusted quite well. But nuisances still remain: lack of adequate dressing rooms in operating suites; limited dormitory facilities; and other obstacles to be overcome.

Other frustrations can also be serious: Few women medical students escape being called, in error, nurse, secretary, or dietitian, by patients and even colleagues. Undoubtedly, over the next few years, women students will continue to face these prejudices as we attempt to overcome society's image that women are not physicians. Surely, as the number of women in the profession increases, and with time, the image will change. Certain male medical students still need to change their attitudes about women. Fortunately women in medical school are finding men less hostile. Women struggle with their desire to be professionally no different from men, yet they do not want to abandon their identity as women.

As a woman applicant, it might be helpful for you to seek out other women currently enrolled on campuses you visit. Try to discover how easily or difficultly adjustments have been made by others. Certainly, if an office for women exists, it demonstrates a certain degree of commitment by the school to help women succeed. It also might be prudent to learn whether there is a good percentage of female faculty. If so, there may be a chance that the school's admissions committee will also have some women as members.

Minority Applicants

In the 1970s, medical school started to make significant and important efforts to recruit and retain minority students. The movement has been successful, in part, but it is still evolving. Some schools have not lived up to their social obligation and are woefully behind. In the early 1970s, the minority applicant pool was extremely low. It peaked in the early 1980s and is now decreasing. It is not altogether clear why; but, certainly, the continued high cost of medical education plays a role. Other less expensive educational alternatives may be drawing minority students away from medicine. And, no doubt, the overall decline in minorities in higher education has had its effect. Government policies no longer offer as much encouragement as they once did. Still, minority students would do well to talk with currently enrolled medical students and recent graduates. They may discover that the personal satisfactions and rewards of a medical career more than offset the time, work, and cost of a medical education. What's more, it is absolutely clear that there is a need for an increased number of minorities in the medical profession.

As a general rule, admissions committees consider a variety of factors in determining an applicant's acceptance into medical school. While GPAs and MCAT scores are used as significant indicators, they are not the only guides. Schools have always reviewed other elements in a student's background. Most schools want a diverse student population. They select students from various areas of the country with various backgrounds, and from different colleges. They try to balance the student body, accepting some from rural settings and others from urban areas. Minority recruitment is just another facet of the selection process.

Minority applicants should be aware that there are special preparatory programs designed to help some who may have experienced educational disadvantage. Many students have found these effective and have successfully entered medical school following these training programs. Good work at such summer programs may be viewed favorably by admissions committee members.

I strongly recommend that you, as a minority student, apply to and select those schools that officially minimize the identification of the minority student group. Of course, you should seek out those schools that support minority efforts to develop and profit from their own political and cultural student associations. But in my opinion, if at all possible, do not look to those schools that offer a special minority educational track. While this may sound contradictory, it isn't. A formal, separate admissions process or educational program for minority students is quite different from the need for minority students to establish and encourage their own identity on campus.

Seek out other minority students enrolled in medical schools. They are an invaluable source of information, providing insight into campus life, attitudes, and other critical factors. Their experiences with their own discomfort or with the prejudices of faculty, peers, and patients will help guide your own decisions.

Your acceptance into medical school should not carry with it an obligation for you to commit yourself to practice in any specific area or with any special population. As a minority student, you will be confronted with faculty, administrators, even your peers, who support your recruitment because minority communities need physicians. Certainly the need is great and urgent, but there is no principal reason why you should assume that responsibility. In my opinion you should approach your medical studies with the same open-minded attitude as all other students who seek careers that best suit their style, personality, and long-range interests. You should have the same choice to practice what you want and where you want to, according to your own desires. In the end you may decide to practice medicine by returning to your community. But that decision should come from the dictates of your own conscience, not from the expectations or demands of others.

In recent years the medical profession has begun to overcome its historic resistance to minorities in its ranks. Undoubtedly, as more minorities emerge from medical schools and as we continue to support and encourage minorities in medicine, the trend will continue. Your acceptance to medical school is another step in that direction.

Detailed information about each school's effort to recruit and maintain minority students can be obtained from the medical schools of your choice. It is also wise to obtain a copy of "Minority Student Opportunities in United States Medical Schools." To order it, write to:

Association of American Medical Colleges
Membership and Publication Orders
Suite 200
One Dupont Circle, N.W.
Washington, DC 20036.

Minority students may list themselves with the Medical Minority Applicant Registry (Med-MAR), a program that automatically sends, without charge, your biographical data to admissions offices throughout the U.S. If you are a black American, Mexican-American, Native American, mainland Puerto Rican, or an applicant from a low-income family, you may complete a special questionnaire to enter the Med-MAR registry when you take your MCAT. Upon reviewing these lists, schools may contact you directly to obtain more information about your application. For details, write to:

Minority Student Information Clearinghouse
Association of American Medical Colleges
One Dupont Circle, N.W.
Washington, DC 20036.

Many minority applicants are in need of financial aid, above that required by most students. Review Chapter 8, "Your Finances," carefully, especially those sections dealing with scholarships and other assistance. Many schools are committed to enrolling minority students and applicants from families with insufficient resources. If you are eager to enter medical school but are afraid that you may not be able to marshal sufficient funds to cover your medical education, you should make every effort to seek financial aid from your school and other sources. If you are a qualified applicant, it is likely that you will be able to assemble enough money, in loans and scholarships, to support your education.

Handicapped Applicants

Opportunities in employment and education for the handicapped are more available than ever before. Many schools have made major efforts to make life on campus more comfortable and accessible to the handicapped. Large numbers of classrooms and dormitory facilities have been restructured, and many recreational facilities have been altered to accommodate students with limited mobility, hearing, or vision.

While medical schools have also joined in this effort, they are faced with special dilemmas in opening medical education to handicapped candidates. There is no doubt that the handicapped need to be encouraged and helped, but medicine as a career for some raises certain critical issues about basic physical requirements demanded of doctors. While access to educational opportunities cannot and should not be restricted on the basis of handicapped status, fundamental questions—which until now have been dealt with only superficially—remain unsettled: Should certain traditional requirements for a medical degree be waived if they cannot be met because of a physical handicap? Should fellow students and faculty be expected to contribute their time and effort for handicapped students who cannot perform certain duties? Do particular handicaps limit potential professional competence or endanger the safety of future patients?

Obviously medical students are expected to perform essential work requiring sight, hearing, and manual dexterity—examining patients, drawing blood, performing invasive diagnostic tests, assisting in surgery, reading X-rays, and listening to patients.

Medicine has not yet come to grips with the problems raised by handicapped medical-school applicants. By tradition and also because of the evaluative methods employed by National Board examinations, graduation from medical school is tantamount to getting a license to practice. With this in mind medical schools grant degrees not only on the basis of whether students meet the requirements for graduation but also based upon whether they ought to be allowed to practice. This is unique to medicine and is not a practice shared by other professions. For instance, when an English teacher decides whether to pass or fail a student taking a particular course, the professor does not worry about whether the student ought to consider an alternative career, even if the student's work is adequate. Law schools confer law degrees and leave access to the practice of law to the bar exam. In all other fields academic accomplishment is separated from certification to practice. If you are handicapped and are seeking admission to medical school, you must certainly be aware that many of these issues will be on the minds of people charged with the responsibility of making decisions about your application. You should give serious thought to these questions and be prepared to offer cogent and resourceful responses to challenges as well as to sincere concerns that surely will be raised.

There is a great need for the handicapped to become physicians. Beyond the moral imperative to offer the handicapped fair and equal access to all opportunities, they bring special insight and understanding, offering important, positive influences to the profession.

White Male Applicants

Until quite recently, medical schools and, consequently, the entire profession itself, was almost entirely a white male preserve. While this group still dominates—as it does most of the powerful institutions in the country—its hold is lessening. Some practicing physicians and certain faculty members are still reluctant to welcome students and doctors from groups outside of their own. A minority of white male students, too, continue to express negative attitudes about other medical students who have only recently been introduced.

Enlightened members of the medical profession and administrators at most schools are making serious efforts to turn the tide. Male/female and white/minority ratios at a good number of institutions reflect the new trend with hitherto underrepresented students receiving larger shares of the total student population. Some white male students who come from privileged or isolated backgrounds may be introduced to students from other ethnic and economic spheres for the first times in their lives. Such students will need to inspect their attitudes and come to terms with their bias. Like it or not, they will be working and studying side-by-side with other highly motivated, well-qualified students of different backgrounds. Some may be unnerved to discover that many of these other students will be sharper than they are.

Just as you must be prepared to face the drama of death, the arduous task of absorbing huge quantities of information, and undergoing other new experiences at medical school, you must also be prepared to share your medical education—and possibly your dorm—with people who may at first seem quite apart. If you are open-minded, you will learn how to live in this new environment. You may even emerge as a mature physician, not only because you learned to deal with the traditional medical school curriculum and its clinical demands but also because you discovered that you can broaden your views about others. If you learn these lessons well, you will be a much better doctor and a sounder human being. Your future patients—of all backgrounds, ages, sexes, and standards of living—will surely appreciate what you have become.

Foreign Applicants

Given the stiff competition for places in American medical schools, foreign applicants don't usually have much of a chance. When you add the fact that most schools give first priority to in-state students, few, if any, spots are open for applicants from other countries. Last year, nearly 400 foreign students applied for admission to U.S. schools. Just slightly over 100 were accepted. Remember that, in all, close to 17,000 students were admitted to U.S. medical schools that year.

Against these odds, it may be best not to try. But, if you are a foreign student and you insist, here are some suggestions: First, get yourself accepted to an undergraduate college in the U.S. Successful applicants from abroad have usually finished one or more years in a U.S. college. Next, make sure your English-language skills are more than just passable. Medical schools may require that you show evidence of superior knowledge of English by passing special examinations. And, finally, be prepared to show that you can afford to pay for your medical education. You may be required to draw up a detailed financial plan, itemizing exactly how you or your family will support you. And don't expect financial aid. Precious little is available for foreign students. Foreign students are not eligible for U.S. federal support.

7.
Rejection

If You're Not Accepted—What Next?

Since luck plays a good part in whether or not you are successful in being admitted to medical school, you should be aware that you are not alone. Thousands of highly qualified, well-motivated students fail to be admitted every year. It is sad, but true, that you are probably as well suited to a medical career as those who are accepted. In many cases it's just the throw of the dice. Competition is fierce, and your chances are modest if you are an average applicant. You may still be left out, even if your credentials are superior.

So what comes next, after you wipe your eyes? If you're intellectually gifted—as many applicants certainly are—you might consider alternative careers in allied sciences, which will give you the opportunity to explore exciting studies in neighboring fields, such as pharmacology, biochemistry, neurobiology, molecular biology, and dozens of other active scientific disciplines. Many of the most striking advances in medical sciences in our day have come from research workers who do not hold medical degrees but who have penetrated the fascinating core of cells, tissues, and genes.

If scientific research is not for you, and you are among those whose interest in medicine is in part due to your desire to work closely with people, there are many careers in which you can demonstrate your interpersonal skills rewardingly for you and for others. Consider clinical psychology, for example. Or opportunities in social services or law.

If your desire to enter medicine was motivated largely by your wish to offer health care to others, you may still have a chance to participate by considering careers in allied health-care professions as a nurse, for instance, or nurse practitioner, physician assistant, midwife, physical therapist, optometrist, dentist, pharmacist, podiatrist, or other critical and highly skilled professions.

Or you may wish to enter neighboring fields where you will work side by side with physicians and others in health-care settings: perhaps as a hospital administrator or in medical or radiation technology.

Don't forget that before you thought about medical school there may have been other things you had in mind. Or you may be highly skilled in totally unrelated fields. You may be remarkably good in theater arts or as a computer programmer. Don't abandon these other interests; they may turn out to be rewarding.

Perhaps your failure to gain admission to medical

school was caused by poor planning and inappropriate choices. It may be helpful for you to go back over the advice given in this handbook to review how you went about it. There may have been a number of things you failed to recognize or did not do right. For example, your MCAT scores may have been not nearly good enough. Or your GPA at college just didn't measure up. Many other factors may have contributed to your lack of success; you may have prepared a poorly formulated or sloppy personal statement; or uninspiring letters of recommendation were submitted. What's worse, you may have filed late or failed to follow critical instructions.

In filing your applications you may have chosen too few schools or not the right ones—perhaps those which did not match your credentials or perhaps others where you could hardly have expected to be accepted. For instance, you may have applied to some schools that accept few out-of-state students, in which case your chances were overwhelmingly small.

In the end you may be among those who unhappily discover that luck had little to do with it. After reviewing what went wrong, you may learn that there was little hope that you would be accepted—your academic and other skills were just not sufficient to warrant entering the race.

Soon after you receive your rejection notice, it might be good for you to look deeply into your soul and ask yourself some tough questions.

"Was I really good enough to get in?" You may find that you secretly knew all along that your record was borderline at best, in which case you never really had a chance, did you?

"Did I really want to get in?" Some students, even with top qualifications, trap themselves into believing that

medical school is destined for them. If you are among them, you may have secretly resisted, sabatoging your chances along the way, getting filing dates mixed up, choosing the wrong schools, flubbing the interview, among other damaging things. You may be relieved to find that you won't have to go to medical school, after all—a place you may have dreaded privately. What's more, you may have forced yourself to apply, not for your own career goals but because your father or your mother was so eager for you to be a doctor. Now that it's over, you can get on with your own life, perhaps fulfilling your own dreams rather than your parents'.

"Am I really right for medicine?" Granted, your desire to get into medical school is real and is your own. Perhaps it even may have been a goal you set for yourself during childhood. But your interviewer and admissions committee members may have picked up something about your motivation and your aims that prevented them from believing that you would succeed in medical school or that you would make a good doctor. A fine academic record, coupled with excellent recommendations and even out-standing extracurricular activities, can still be a screen behind which you hide the sad fact that your only true goal was *getting into medical school*. Beyond that, you may not have given any serious thought to medicine or to your future career as a doctor. And this may have come through.

But, if after you've looked into your soul you still think that you are a good candidate, but fate blocked your way or perhaps some technical goof spoiled your chances, by all means reapply.

Reapplying

Students who have not been successful in gaining admission to medical school and who do not wish (or cannot afford) to go to a foreign medical school may reapply the following year. Since the quality of the applicant pool has remained relatively stable over a number of years, it is safe to say that those who were previously rejected will be rejected again. But remember that luck will once again be a factor. The second time, fate may offer a different outcome. Obviously this is true for reasonably well-qualified applicants. Luck does not rescue a poor candidate.

Certainly evidence of continued study and improved performance on your next MCAT will greatly enhance your chances. New letters of recommendation, based on current activities, might also contribute. And, of course, one should certainly consider applying to new schools. Caution: Almost all applications will ask you if you have applied before. As a previous applicant, your name will appear on rosters of prior-year applicants—so be honest.

Foreign Medical Schools

Sadly, many unsuspecting students, and others who should know better, turn in desperation to certain schools abroad where the quality of teaching is modest at best, criminally negligent at worst.

There are a number of high-quality medical schools in other countries, comparable to, or even better than, some in the U.S. But these institutions, largely in Western

Europe (but also elsewhere), rarely accept students from the U.S. Most, if not all, of their students come from their home countries. If you're lucky enough to get into one of these quality institutions abroad, very likely you will receive an education on a par with that offered in U.S. schools.

Of course, Canadian medical schools are equivalent to U.S. institutions and should not be thought of as "foreign" in the same sense as others in this section. For details about schools in Canada, turn to page 303.

A few years ago Congress investigated some of the profit-making foreign medical schools that encourage U.S. applicants. The report that followed found that the medical education provided was sadly lacking. Not one lived up to the standards of a single U.S. or Canadian medical school. The schools studied had relatively poor facilities, equipment, faculty, and curriculum standards. Worst of all, clinical training was severely limited. None of the foreign schools gave students a sufficient range of clinical facilities or experience.

Private, profit-making medical schools in the Caribbean and elsewhere in Latin American and other parts of the world use enticing ads to appeal to candidates who are unsuccessful in getting into U.S. medical schools. Occasionally they play up the fact that U.S. students are eligible to obtain federally guaranteed student loans. The implication is that these schools are somehow approved of in the U.S. But just because you can get a loan backed by the federal government is no endorsement of the school's quality or acceptability.

If you're thinking about going abroad to one of the schools that exploit the desire of many Americans to get a medical degree, no matter what, be aware that if you go, your chances of emerging as a fairly ignorant physician are pretty good. And for this privilege be prepared to pay handsomely. Application fees are high and tuition is very expensive. Plus there is no guarantee that you will ever be able to practice in the U.S.

"Will I Be Able to Come Back?"

Most students who study medicine abroad seek to complete their education by coming back to the United States, either by gaining admission to a U.S. medical school as a transfer student or by attempting to enter a graduate program here.

Many try to gain admission to U.S. medical schools in their third year—the most likely and frequent entry point— but their chances are still slim. Very few places are ever open. What's more, most schools require that transfer students take a stiff exam, known as the Medical Sciences Knowledge Profile (MSKP). The test is given in June every year, and applicants must register about two months in advance. For information write to:

MSKP, Division of Student Services
Association of American Medical Colleges
1776 Massachusetts Avenue, N.W., Suite 301
Washington, DC 20036-1989
(202) 828-0603.

Others seek to gain admission to U.S. graduate programs, after they complete their studies abroad. But it's not easy. They must first be accepted by the Accreditation

Council of Graduate Medical Education (ACGME) and then pass a special test, known as Foreign Medical Graduates Examination in the Medical Sciences (FMGEMS). Usually given in July, the two-day exam tests your knowledge of basic sciences on the first day and covers your clinical experience and skills on the next. Both aliens and U.S. citizens who graduate from foreign medical schools are required to pass the exam to be eligible for admission to accredited residency or fellowship programs in the U.S.

Even if you are fortunate enough to receive accreditation and you pass the FMGEMS exam, you should be aware that few places are likely to be open to you. Right now the number of students who graduate from U.S. medical schools is almost equal to the number of postgraduate residencies available. Chances are that foreign-trained graduates will have little likelihood of being accepted in a postgraduate program in this country and practically no possibility of being admitted into highly competitive specialties.

Commercial Services: A Warning

You may also come across ads for companies that claim to help—even guarantee—admission to medical schools abroad. Some services suggest that they can assist you in gaining acceptance at U.S. medical schools. But be warned: These unscrupulous firms offer no more help than you can get from consulting your own pre-med adviser or from reading this handbook or other similar publications. In the bargain, such services charge fees that can run into hundreds of thousands of dollars.

8.
Your
Finances

Your medical education will cost a considerable amount of money. This chapter will not attempt to diminish the truth of that statement, but it may help you to realize that it may be a financial burden worth taking on. While the costs are great, intelligent planning and a modest amount of sophistication in coming to terms with money matters may help to reduce your anxiety about assuming so large a debt. Remember that in return for your investment you will be receiving the benefits of a medical education, so it pays to consider the financial questions carefully.

Once you have been accepted to a medical school, the best thing to do is to learn about financial aid and other money matters from the school directly. You'll find out what is offered, what plans and loans are available. Your financial-aid office will provide you with brochures, catalogs, and other materials. Study these items closely.

You'll come to appreciate that there are two principal types of aid. If you can get it, the first is surely best—gift support (scholarships, grants, and tuition refunds). The other source—loans—require that you eventually pay back what you borrow, almost always with interest. In addition, there are a few programs that require that you provide medical service, after you complete your M.D., in exchange for financial support for your training.

About 80 percent of all students in medical school receive some form of financial help. Still, all schools believe that you and your family must assume primary responsibility for meeting your medical-school financial obligation. When you are accepted, ask your school to provide you with their current estimates of all costs—not only tuition and fees but also all living costs.

"Can I Afford It?"

The cost of a medical education can vary considerably, depending on whether you are accepted into a school in your state or by a private medical school. At the low end are California's state schools, with current annual costs for residents running at approximately $1,500. The most expensive are schools such as the University of Colorado where annual tuition for out-of-state students is approximately $26,800.

In addition to tuition and fees, the cost of living also varies by geographic area. Living costs can play a major part in your total budget: room and board, books, equipment, travel, personal needs, and entertainment, among other things. Of course, students who depend upon financial aid do not live in an elegant style, but your budget should include enough to have a little bit of fun.

Keep in mind that while some catalogs list tuition as free, fees can be large. Historically and for special reasons, tuition and fees are listed separately. But you should be aware that it is the *total* cost of tuition—plus fees and living costs—that determines the actual amount of money that you will need to come up with. In the directory at the end of this handbook is a list of each U.S. and Canadian school giving annual tuition, fees, and projected estimated living costs for all students.

Financing

Students, mostly unsophisticated about money, frequently are overwhelmed by the total cost of their education, especially when it's calculated on a ten- or twenty-year repayment schedule. For example, a $10,000 loan at 11 percent, repaid over 15 years, will come to a total repayment of $20,500. The business world considers this an acceptable, fair price to pay for the long-term use of someone else's money.

It might be helpful to look at it this way: If you need financial aid, think about what most people do when buying a home. Nearly everyone takes out a mortgage. Consider the purchase of an $80,000 home for people with a $10,000 down payment. They'll have a $70,000 mortgage, say, at 12 percent interest over 30 years. When they finish, they'll have paid a total of $259,200. Is this excessive? It all depends. The alternative is not being able to buy the home they want with the cash they have available.

The most important consideration for these home-buyers, and for you as a medical student, is not the *size* of the loan but the *terms and repayment schedule*. People who take out a loan must determine if they can manage to cover their monthly payments based on their expected future income. If you do this calculation correctly, you'll learn whether or not you will be fiscally solvent or go broke during the first ten or fifteen years following medical school. Over the long haul most people conclude that taking out a mortgage on a home is a worthwhile investment. Financing your medical education is considered just as good—if not better—a deal by most students.

As you feel the joy and heave a sigh of relief over your acceptance to medical school, a nagging question emerges: "Can I afford it?" Will you be able to generate the necessary financial resources? You'll also wonder, "How much aid will I get from the school?"

Eligibility for Financial Aid

While no two schools offer the same financial package, some common concepts are used. It's important that you understand them. The first question is: Are you eligible for financial aid? Most schools offer financial aid to students based on *demonstrated* and *verified* need. A few offer inducements (or merit scholarships), independent of demonstrated financial need. Which schools offer these scholarships and how much they give change from year to year. School catalogs and financial-aid booklets publish the extent, criteria, and amount of aid offered. As you'd expect, merit scholarships are given to students with exceptional academic records and are awarded to a very small percentage of students.

Needs Analysis

Virtually all students who receive aid, either directly from their school or indirectly from a bank (after authorization by the school), must undergo a "needs analysis." Needs analyses assess all of the resources you can call upon to finance your medical education—your personal resources plus that of your family and, if you are married, your spouse. Frequently these assessments are performed by outside private agencies, such as the Graduate and Professional School Financial Aid Service (GAPSFAS), the College Scholarship Service (CSS), the American College Testing (ACT) Program, or by the school's independent needs analysis system.

These services review your entire financial picture: money in the bank, stocks, bonds, property, homes, investments, debts, liens, taxes, etc. They will consider other factors, such as other siblings in school, your age, your parents' imminent or current retirement, family medical bills, employment. In the end they will judge how much money they will expect you or your family to contribute annually. If this amount equals or exceeds what your school expects you to pay, you will not be eligible for aid. If, however, they determine that your annual medical-school bill exceeds your resources, your school will offer you some form of financial aid.

Currently you should assume that a good share, if not most, of your demonstrated need will be met by loans. If your need is so great that it exceeds certain basic amounts set by the school, additional funds may then be met by scholarships, if funds are available. Each school has its own formula to determine how much it will allow you to borrow and how much it will provide in scholarships. Many schools employ what is called a "unit" or "base" loan, requiring you to take out an initial amount in loans. If your need exceeds this amount, additional scholarships are made available. While this is a very common practice, not all schools follow this procedure. What's more, a large number of combinations and permutations of loan/scholarship ratios exist. Loans and scholarship plans change annually, depending on resources available at each school. It's best to consult the financial-aid office or school catalog for details.

"Need," as viewed by most institutions, is not an amount of money that the school feels it is legally or morally committed to offer. "If funds are available" is always a caveat at the back of your financial-aid brochure. Still, most schools feel a deep obligation to offer as much as they can to meet your needs and to help you get the rest from other sources. Your financial aid officer will assist you, and the school's brochure will list many sources for which you may be eligible.

Federal Support

During the last decade the U.S. government has made available a considerable amount of money to students to help finance their medical education. Before you go any further, you should know what is available. The government-sponsored programs listed here give information as of early 1985. But before you apply it's best to check with your financial-aid office and your local bank to make sure qualifications, rates, and other details are in effect.

Guaranteed Student Loans (GSL)

These loans allow you to borrow directly from your local bank, school, credit union, savings and loan association, or other lending institution. They are administered by various state agencies, and so they are often called "state loans." States and lenders set their own policies regarding how much they offer and to whom, so it's not easy to predict exactly what you will encounter when you seek a GSL loan. To qualify you must show that your family income is not sufficient to support your medical education or that you qualify because of need. To determine whether your situation fits these criteria, you must complete and submit a Guaranteed Student Loan Needs Test form, together with an Application for a Guaranteed Student Loan.

Family Income. You will quality for a GSL on the basis of "family income," if your family's adjusted gross income is less than $30,000.

Financial Need. If your family's adjusted gross income is greater than $30,000 and your school determines that you still require a loan to meet the cost of your education, you may qualify for a GSL on the basis of "financial need." The U.S. Department of Education sets the guideline for how your school calculates how much your family is expected to contribute. Your family's expected contribution, plus all other sources of aid, are added together. If this total doesn't meet the cost of your education, you may qualify.

When you apply for these loans, you must submit supporting income documentation. A tax return is sufficient, but if none was filed, you must provide other income evidence. In either case, these items must be submitted to your financial-aid office, together with your federally approved needs analysis application, which is available from your financial-aid officer.

Guaranteed Student Loans are currently at 8 percent interest. While you are in school the government pays the interest for you. Afterward, during the "repayment period," you are required to pay back the principal. You are allowed to borrow up to $5,000 per year, but your total for all years cannot exceed $25,000. At this moment, this limit also includes any loans you may have obtained as an undergraduate. Further limits are likely, as the government cuts back on loans.

The government permits your local bank to charge you—in addition to interest—an "origination" fee of 5 percent of the total amount you borrow from them. Your state's Student Loan Foundation also charges an insurance fee, deducted from your loan before you receive it. Check with your bank for details.

If you took out a Guaranteed Student Loan to help finance your college education and your interest then was at 7 percent, if you borrow again under the GSL program for medical school, interest on your new loan will also be at 7 percent. You will also be entitled to a nine-month "grace" period; that is, you'll have an extra nine months after you graduate from medical school to start repayment. Similarly, if you previously borrowed money under this program at 9 percent, your current loan will remain at 9 percent; but instead of a nine-month grace period, you will have six months after graduation before you must start to repay the loan. The six-month grace period also applies to loans for students whose earlier GSL was at 8 percent. These new loans, just like the earlier ones, also remain at 8 percent.

The repayment period usually runs from five to ten years but deferments of up to three years are permitted for those who join the armed forces, Peace Corps, or VISTA—or if you become an officer in the U.S. Public Health Service. Other deferments are available for students who are temporarily or totally disabled. What's more, all students may usually defer payments for up to two years during their medical residency.

Health Professions Student Loans (HPSL)

This program is designed for students who are in "exceptional" financial need, whose total available resources do not exceed $5,000. Schools select those who qualify by assessing their financial situation in the light of a national need-analysis system. The school also reviews other information about students' financial status, including any contributions likely to come from parents, themselves, or—if married—their spouse.

The maximum amount available per year is tuition plus $2,500. But since each school has limited funds for the program, qualified students usually receive much less than the maximum. The interest rate is at 9 percent, and both principal and interest repayment is deferred until after residency training or if you perform military or Peace Corps service. This loan provides a twelve-month grace period and is to be paid back over ten years. Interest accrues on the unpaid balance when you start paying the loan.

National Direct Student Loans (NDSL)

Given on the basis of need, these loans provide a maximum of $12,000, including any loans made to the student before entering graduate or professional school. The loan offers a six-month grace period and the interest rate is 5 percent. Upon graduation from medical school you may defer payment for up to two years while you are a resident. Deferred payments of up to three years are available to students entering the Peace Corps, VISTA, the military, or public health service. Extensions are also available for disabled students. Commonly the repayment period is ten years.

Auxiliary Loans to Assist Students Program (ALAS) or Parental Loans to Undergraduate Students (PLUS)

Under this program graduate and professional students may borrow up to $3,000 per year, as long as they are at least half-time students. No student may borrow more than $15,000 from this source. While it does not carry a loan "origination" fee, there is an insurance fee, deducted before payment is made. Current interest rate is 12 percent and will remain constant throughout the life of the loan.

Because this loan is not subsidized, interest will begin to accrue from the start. You may even be required to pay interest monthly or quarterly while you are in school, but the principal may be deferred as long as you are enrolled at least part-time. No grace period is offered, and you must pay a minimum of $50 per month. You have up to ten years to repay, but you are entitled to defer the principal for up to two years during the period you are a resident.

Health Education Assistance Loans (HEAL)

This is a nonsubsidized loan program where eligible medical students may borrow up to $20,000 per year, up to a total of $80,000. Interest is usually calculated at a variable rate—using the 91-day Treasury bill rate as a base plus 3.5 percent—compounded semiannually. Repayment begins twelve months after you cease to be a full-time student. As a resident, you may defer payment for up to four years. You have from ten to twenty-five years (excluding deferment periods) to repay. A three-year extension on payments is also permitted for those who join the military, Peace Corps, National Health Service Corps, or VISTA. Ask your financial-aid office for details.

Shrinking Federal Support

Recently, funds for these programs have eroded. Some project that still further cuts will be made in federally sponsored loans. No one knows whether Congress will permit the decline to continue at the same rapid rate. But make no mistake: Do not expect the amount of money available to support medical students to increase.

"Good" vs. "Bad" Money

Not fully appreciated by most prospective borrowers is a consideration of "good" vs. "bad" money. "Good" money is low-interest, subsidized, deferred-payment loans; "bad" money is high-interest, immediate-payment, nondeferrable loans. Interest rates and payback schedules can make a big difference to you when it comes time to make your monthly payments when your loans come due. It's best to obtain a schedule of your projected monthly payments for each loan over the life of its entire repayment period. You'll be in a better position to understand the financial obligation you have assumed.

Your financial-aid officer is governed by federal regulations when setting limits on the amount you will be permitted to borrow from each loan program. Very likely you will borrow money to finance your medical education from three or more sources. Each loan will have a different interest rate, grace period, deferment option, and duration of repayment. You can project what your financial burden will be over the life of your loans to help you assess your future obligations.

Remember that interest paid on student loans, like interest paid on mortgages, will be deductible from your future income-tax reports. Do not feel that this is an unimportant consideration. It may make the difference when you measure your projected future income against what you will be required to repay. You'll then be better able to decide whether you will have enough left over to put food on your table.

When you evaluate financial aid "packages" (the term used for all loans and scholarships combined), pursue loans that are in the "good money" category and shy away, if possible, from the "bad money."

Also keep in mind when calculating your budget and taking out a loan that the face value of the loan may not be equal to the amount of money you will actually get. Charges, deductions, and other so-called "front-loading" costs may turn a $5,000 loan into one as low as $4,500 to put in your pocket.

Interest and Rates

Interest rates on your loans can be quite varied—simple, compound, subsidized, accrued, or variable. "Simple interest" is a *fixed* percentage on the original money you borrowed. "Compound interest" continuously applies the interest due for each pay period to the sum of your original loan and adds that amount over the previous interest period. "Subsidized interest" loans are the best, of course, because your school or the government pays the interest for you. You have no obligation to pay the interest while you are in school. This means that the original money you borrowed will remain the same until repayment starts. Recently, "variable-interest" loans have been applied to student loans in a manner similar to variable-interest mortgages. Under these conditions the rate charged fluctuates with Treasury bill rates or with some other monitor of the money market.

Applying for Financial Aid

In addition to requiring a needs analysis by an outside independent agency, most schools will ask you to submit a number of other documents to determine and verify your financial situation. Be prepared to fill out an extensive application and to document it with copies of IRS forms, birth certificates for children, marriage licenses, adoption papers, etc.

At the time of your interview, do not hesitate to seek out information from the school's financial-aid office and obtain a copy of their financial-aid booklet. It will not jeopardize your chances. Most schools anticipate that a very high percentage of students will require some form of financial aid. They do not allow the financial status of students to influence their decision.

Are You an Independent Student?

While all students would like to be considered "independent" and frequently have disassociated themselves from family financial ties in order to qualify for IRS definitions of independence, at medical school they discover that their "independence" is not accepted for certain types of financial assistance. While each school sets its own guidelines, and a few schools will accept your professed financial independence, most schools will not accept your statement of independence for some federal loan programs, even if you are eligible to be declared independent by federal standards.

Schools that do not accept your independence will require that your family and/or spouse participate in a needs-analysis test. Exceptions to the rule are the GSL, ALAS, and HEAL funds. If you can meet the federal definition of independence, you may qualify for these loans.

Additional Sources of Support

Most students become rapidly familiar with the major sources that are available to all students. But there are also large numbers of grants that are available to students exhibiting specific criteria, such as their place of birth, college, particular medical school, career objectives, etc. Most financial-aid offices will have booklets listing a large number of foundations, societies, and other agencies with money available. Generally these are small amounts, but they can make an important contribution if you are eligible. Your school may also have special funds designed for you. Check with your financial-aid office.

You may also wish to consider the following programs.

Armed Forces Health Professions Scholarship Program offers a medical education free of charge to those willing to commit themselves to a significant number of years of military service after earning their degree. Various branches of the armed forces (the army, navy, and air force) offer scholarships to students attending private or public schools with the understanding that for each year of financial support (which includes tuition and a stipend) the student will commit one year to military service. You are also required to serve forty-five days of active duty for annual training.

For more information about these military-supported scholarships, write to these addresses. For the army: Commander, Army Medical Department Personnel Support Agency, Department of the Army, Attn: SGPE-PDM-S, 1900 Half Street, S.W., Washington, D.C. 20314; or call collect, (202) 693-5120. The navy's program is at: Naval Medical Command, Code 554, Department of the Navy, Washington, D.C. 20372. And for the air force write: Headquarters, USAF Recruiting Service, Directorate of Health Professions Recruiting, Randolph AFB, TX 78150. The toll-free number is (800) 531-5980.

The National Health Service Corps, currently being phased out, offered tuition and stipends for those who would work in areas designated by the Secretary of NHS.

There are a few combined M.D./Ph.D. programs sponsored by the Medical Scientist Training Program of the National Institutes of Health, which gives a stipend and tuition for six or seven years (see page 104).

Scholarship Program for First-year Students of Exceptional Financial Need. Open to students who demonstrate "exceptional" financial need, this scholarship provides tuition plus some funds for other educational expenses. You need not provide any service upon graduation in exchange for the tuition reimbursement or stipend. Consult your financial-aid office for details. But remember that funds are quite limited and only the most in need will be eligible.

National Medical Fellowships (NMF). Designed especially for underrepresented minority students—Native Americans, mainland Puerto Ricans, Mexican Americans, and blacks. For further information write to: Scholarship Program, National Medical Scholarships, Inc., Room 1820, 250 West 57 Street, New York, NY 10107.

State Programs. In addition, some states offer forgiveness loans if you agree to practice for a stipulated period of time in that state. A financial-aid package is provided, giving the usual amount of loans. Once you commit yourself to practice in the state, your loans are canceled. These programs change quite frequently, so inquire about them from your financial-aid office.

Employment

There's little doubt that working while you are in medical school is very difficult. Few students are fortunate enough to possess skills that are much in demand and for which they can obtain a significant amount of money. Working to pay your way through medical school competes with your schedule and may undermine your education. Most schools discourage employment and try to arrange enough of a financial-aid package to meet your minimal requirements for getting through without work. What's more, work may backfire in other ways: If you become gainfully employed, many schools add that income into your total resources when they calculate your financial need.

Repayment

After graduation you will have to face repaying your loans.
If you're lucky, most of your loans will have a grace period
and a deferment, which, when added together, will postpone the beginning of your monthly installments for up to
three to five years. If some of your obligations are "bad-
money" loans, you may have to start paying as early as two
months after graduation.

*Will you be fiscally solvent during the height of your
repayment schedule?* Graduates of medical schools in June
1985 entered postgraduate training receiving an average
salary of $22,000 a year. At the completion of their resi-
dency program (depending on whether it is for three or
five years) salaries are likely to rise to about $28,000.
Depending on their career choice, they will enter a
practice and/or assume responsibility as an employed physician at salaries considerably higher than that.

If most of your loans are deferred throughout residency training, and repayment begins when you are
employed as a physician, you are likely to be fiscally
solvent. Problems arise for those students who, because of
larger than usual indebtedness, caused, perhaps, by family or other extraordinary expenses, may find repayment a
burden.

Must you repay your loans? The government's argument for cutting down on student-loan appropriations,
apart from cutting government spending in general, comes
from the disclosure that, unfortunately, certain students
have felt no obligation to repay their loans. Legislators
end up feeling that high-income physicians certainly ought
to repay the taxpayers for the use of their money. Your

access to federal funds for your medical education is being hurt by those who have tried to get away without repaying. The government intends to crack down on those who fail to repay their loans. Be advised that your loans are contractual commitments with all the legal obligations and penalties associated with a binding contract.

Your Role

Medical schools are eager and willing to help you finance your education. They go a long way to keep your financial situation out of the picture when they decide on whether to admit you. Often schools are frustrated in their ability to help students who feel that the school owes them not only financial support but a very good standard of living too. Often aid officers are not pleased—and rightly so—by students who complain about doing the paperwork, verifying resources, supplying family data, and the other procedures.

Many of the strict rules, requirements for certain forms and documentation, and the need to provide copies of IRS tax forms are caused by blatantly unethical student maneuvers designed to increase financial aid to the undeserving. Misrepresentation of resources, unstated assets, and other false statements have forced schools to police the financial-award system. Obviously all this has become unpleasant for many students. The introduction of a "needs-analysis" and the requirement that you provide IRS documentation is an effort to institute uniform and fair procedures in allocating funds for all.

In the end the responsibility is yours. Even though your school is willing to help, you must shoulder some of the responsibility. So be cooperative, and above all, be honest.

9.
Directory of
U.S. and
Canadian
Medical
Schools

How to Use the Directory

These listings provide you with capsule descriptions of 124 medical schools in the U.S., 3 in Puerto Rico, and 16 in Canada. U.S. schools are given in alphabetical order by state (with entries for Puerto Rico listed among them). Canadian schools follow, in alphabetical order by province. Special Canadian information is given on page 305. Listings open with the name, address, and telephone number for each school.

The data has been compiled from the most reliable sources. But you should be aware that since many items are subject to change—especially financial matters having to do with tuition and other costs—it's wise to contact the schools of your choice, before applying, to receive the latest information.

All U.S. schools offer four-year programs, except for the University of Minnesota at Duluth, with a two-year program. Students there move to the Minneapolis campus to complete their degrees.

Each listing is divided into six sections, under the following headings.

Application and Acceptance. Here you'll find key dates and deadlines. You'll note that some entries have "AMCAS" filing dates, indicating that the school participates in what is known as the American Medical College Application Service. When you apply to these schools, you need only submit one standard application and the service directs copies to all participating schools you select. (For details, turn to page 91.) All other schools request that you send your application to them directly. The phrase "Early Decision Plan" refers to programs available in certain schools whereby students agree to apply early to only one school and to attend that school if they are admitted. (For details see page 101.)

Approximate Expenses per Year. Approximate costs of tuition and fees are given for each school. "Other costs" represent room, board, and other items and are likely to vary for each student, especially if travel to and from home is included.

Statistics. Pay close attention to these figures. This section arms you with data to determine the likelihood of your being admitted. GPA stands for grade-point average. (See page 77 for details.)

Requirements. Offers a brief description of certain items you are required to have performed before you apply.

Required College Courses. Provides a list of undergraduate college courses the school requires that you take before you gain admission. Some colleges have different terminology for similar subjects, so inquire whether the courses you have taken in college are equivalent to those required.

Recommended College Courses. Suggests courses that the school finds helpful but not mandatory.

U.S. Medical Schools

University of Alabama School of Medicine

Director of Admissions
University of Alabama
School of Medicine
Box 318 University Station
Birmingham, AL 35294   Tel: (205) 934-2330

Application and Acceptance (1987–88):
AMCAS application filing: June 15–Nov. 1, 1986
Fee: $25
Offers Early Decision Plan (residents only)
    EDP application filing: June 15–Aug. 1, 1986
    Notification by: Oct. 1, 1986
Regular applicants notified: Dec. 15, 1986–July 1987
Deposit: $50
Estimated new entrants: 150
School starts: July 1987

Approximate Expenses per Year (1985–86):
Tuition: $3,000 (resident); $11,700 (nonresident)
Fees: $1,100
Other costs: $6,600

Statistics (1985–86):
Applicants: 763 (428 in-state; 335 out-of-state)
New entrants: 150 (144 in-state; 6 out-of-state)
Mean GPA: 3.53

Requirements: MCAT, three years of college (90 sem. hrs.), bachelor's degree recommended, preference given to Alabama residents.

Required College Courses: Years
General biology or zoology 1
Chemistry, organic (with lab) 1
        inorganic (with lab) 1
Physics (with lab) 1
Mathematics (incl. calculus) 1
English, composition 1
      literature 1

Recommended College Courses: Behavioral sciences.

University of South Alabama College of Medicine

Office of Admissions
Room 2015, Medical Sciences Building
University of South Alabama
College of Medicine
Mobile, AL 36688   Tel: (205) 460-7176

Application and Acceptance (1987–88):
AMCAS application filing: June 15–Nov. 1, 1986
Fee: $25
Offers Early Decision Plan (residents only)
    EDP application filing: June 15–Aug. 1, 1986
    Notification by: Oct. 1, 1986
Regular applicants notified from: Oct. 15, 1986
Deposit: $50
Estimated new entrants: 64
School starts: Aug. 1987

Approximate Expenses per Year (1985–86):
Tuition: $3,600 (resident); $7,200 (nonresident)
Fees: $700
Other costs: $6,000

Statistics (1985–86):
Applicants: 634 (435 in-state; 199 out-of-state)
New entrants: 65 (63 in-state; 2 out-of-state)
Mean GPA: 3.46

Requirements: MCAT, three years of college (90 sem. hrs.),
    bachelor's degree highly recommended, preference given
    to Alabama residents.

Required College Courses: Sem./Qtr.
General biology (with lab) 2/3
General chemistry (with lab)...2/3
Organic chemistry (with lab) 2/3
General physics (with lab) ....,.2/3
Humanities 2/3
English composition 2/3
Calculus (statistics may be substituted for 1 qtr./1 sem.) 2/3

Recommended College Courses: Quantitative analysis, compar-
    ative vertebrate anatomy, vertebrate embryology, modern
    genetics, and information management (computer science).

University of Arizona College of Medicine

Admissions Office
University of Arizona
College of Medicine
Arizona Health Sciences Center
Tucson, AZ 85724

Tel: (602) 626-6214

Application and Acceptance (1987–88):
AMCAS application filing: June 15–Nov. 1, 1986
Notification from: Jan. 15, 1987
Estimated new entrants: 88
School starts: July 1987

Approximate Expenses per Year (1985–86):
Tuition: $2,700
Other costs: $7,600

Statistics (1985–86):
Applicants: 643 (349 in-state; 294 out-of-state)
New entrants: 88 (87 in-state; 1 out-of-state)
Mean GPA: 3.53
Sex: 38.6% women; 61.4% men

Requirements: MCAT, three years of college (90 sem./135 qtr. hrs.), resident of Arizona or WICHE-certified resident of Alaska, Montana, or Wyoming.

Required College Courses: Sem./Qtr.
General biology or zoology (with lab) 2/3
General chemistry (with lab)..2/3
Organic chemistry (with lab) 2/3
Physics (with lab)..2/3
English 2/3

Recommended College Courses: Social sciences and humanities.

University of Arkansas College of Medicine

Office of Student Admissions, Slot 551
University of Arkansas
College of Medicine
4301 West Markham Street
Little Rock, AR 72205   Tel: (501) 661-5354

Application and Acceptance (1987–88):
AMCAS application filing: June 15–Nov. 15, 1986
Fee: $10
Notification: Dec. 15, 1986–Feb. 15, 1987
Estimated new entrants: 150
School starts: Aug. 1987

Approximate Expenses per Year (1985–86):
Tuition: $3,500 (resident); $7,000 (nonresident)
Fees: $350
Other costs: $6,400

Statistics (1985–86):
Applicants: 441 (298 in-state; 143 out-of-state)
New entrants: 150 (150 in-state; 0 out-of-state)
Mean GPA: 3.6
Sex: 25% women; 75% men

Requirements: MCAT, 90 sem. hrs. college credit (bachelor's
    degree recommended), preference given to Arkansas
    residents.

Recommended College Courses:
Biology (general biology, zoology or botany, genetics, embryology)
Chemistry (general chemistry, organic chemistry)
General physics and mathematics
Behavioral sciences (general or special psychology, sociology,
    ethnology, human ecology, physical or cultural anthropology)
Humanities (English composition, world literature, logic, world
    history, foreign language)

University of California, Davis
School of Medicine

Chair, Admissions Committee
Admissions Office
University of California, Davis
School of Medicine
Davis, CA 95616   Tel: (916) 752-2717

Application and Acceptance (1987–88):
AMCAS application filing: June 15–Nov. 1, 1986
Fee: $35
Notification: Oct. 15, 1986–May 15, 1987
Estimated new entrants: 93
School starts: Sept. 1987

Approximate Expenses per Year (1985–86):
Tuition: $1,700 (resident); $5,300 (nonresident)
Other costs: $9,300

Statistics (1985–86):
Applicants: 3,376 (2,854 in-state; 522 out-of-state)
New entrants: 93 (90 in-state; 3 out-of-state)
Mean GPA: 3.0 minimum

Requirements: MCAT, three years of college (90 sem./135 qtr. hrs.), bachelor's degree recommended, preference given to California residents.

Required College Courses: Years
English 1
Biological science (with lab) 1
General chemistry (with lab) 1
Organic chemistry (with lab) 1
Physics 1
Mathematics (coursework sufficient to satisfy prerequisites
  for integral calculus required)................................1

Recommended College Courses: Biochemistry, genetics, embryology, integral calculus.

University of California, Irvine
California College of Medicine

Office of Admissions
University of California, Irvine
California College of Medicine
Irvine, CA 92717   Tel: (714) 856-5388

Application and Acceptance (1987–88):
AMCAS application filing: June 15–Nov. 15, 1986
Fee: $35
Notification: Nov. 1, 1986–Sept. 1987
Estimated new entrants: 92
School starts: Sept. 1987

Approximate Expenses per Year (1985–86):
Tuition: $1,400 (resident); $5,000 (nonresident)
Other costs: $7,500

Statistics (1985–86):
Applicants: 3,606 (3,031 in-state; 575 out-of-state)
New entrants: 92 (92 in-state; 0 out-of-state)
Mean GPA: 3.6

Requirements: MCAT, three years of college (bachelor's degree recommended), preference given to California residents.

Required College Courses: Years
Biology and/or zoology 1½
Inorganic chemistry 1
Organic chemistry 1
Physics 1
Calculus ....(1 qtr.)

University of California, Los Angeles
UCLA School of Medicine

Office of Student Affairs
Division of Admissions
University of California, Los Angeles
UCLA School of Medicine
Center for Health Sciences
Los Angeles, CA 90024   Tel: (213) 825-6081

Application and Acceptance (1987–88):
AMCAS application filing: June 15–Nov. 1, 1986
Fee: $35
Notification from: Feb. 15, 1987
Estimated new entrants: 140
School starts: Sept. 1987

Approximate Expenses per Year (1985–86):
Tuition: $1,300 (resident); $5,000 (nonresident)
Other costs: $8,000

Statistics (1985–86):
Applicants: 4,233 (2,862 in-state; 1,371 out-of-state)
New entrants: 140 (127 in-state; 13 out-of-state)
Mean GPA: science, 3.6; nonscience, 3.6

Requirements: MCAT, three years of college (bachelor's degree ordinarily required).

Required College Courses: Years
Chemistry (incl. inorganic and organic, quantitative analysis)....2
Biology (incl. cellular, molecular, and developmental
    biology, genetics, and 1 yr. of upper-division courses)....2
Physics (with lab) 1
Mathematics (incl. algebra)...1
English (incl. composition) 1

Recommended College Courses: Physical chemistry, introductory calculus, Spanish.

University of California, San Diego
School of Medicine

Office of Admissions, M-021
Medical Teaching Facility
University of California, San Diego
School of Medicine
La Jolla, CA 92093   Tel: (619) 452-3880

Application and Acceptance (1987–88):
AMCAS application filing: June 15–Nov. 1, 1986
Fee: $35
Notification from: Oct. 15, 1986
Estimated new entrants: 122
School starts: Sept. 1987

Approximate Expenses per Year (1985–86):
Tuition: $1,500 (resident); $4,800 (nonresident)
Other costs: $5,400

Statistics (1985–86):
Applicants: 4,101 (2,882 in-state; 1,219 out-of-state)
New entrants: 122 (114 in-state; 8 out-of-state)
Mean GPA: 3.6
Sex: 26% women; 74% men

Requirements: MCAT, three years of college (bachelor's degree recommended), preference given to California residents.

Required College Courses: Years
Biology (excl. botany)..1
Chemistry (incl. organic)...2
Physics 1
Mathematics (may include calculus, statistics, computer
    science)...1

Recommended College Courses: Behavioral sciences, biology of cells and development, genetics, biochemistry, English (speaking and writing competence), social sciences, conversational Spanish.

University of California, San Francisco
School of Medicine

Admissions Officer
University of California, San Francisco
School of Medicine (S-215)
San Francisco, CA 94143   Tel: (415) 666-4044

Application and Acceptance (1987–88):
AMCAS application filing: June 15–Nov. 1, 1986
Fee: $35
Notification: Dec. 15, 1986–April 15, 1987
Estimated new entrants: 141
School starts: Sept. 1987 (July 1987 for summer enrollment)

Approximate Expenses per Year (1985–86):
Tuition: $1,500 (resident); $5,300 (nonresident)
Fees: $200
Other costs: $7,500

Statistics (1985–86):
Applicants: 4,656 (2,694 in-state; 1,962 out-of-state)
New entrants: 141 (119 in-state; 22 out-of-state)
Mean GPA: 3.69
Sex: 45% women; 55% men

Requirements: MCAT, three years of college (90 sem./135 qtr. hrs.), bachelor's degree strongly recommended, preference given to California residents.

Required College Courses: Years
Biology (incl. vertebrate zoology with lab)....................................1
General chemistry (with lab) 1
Organic chemistry..(2 qtrs.)
Physics (with lab) 1

Recommended College Courses: Mathematics (calculus), upper-division biological sciences, biochemistry, humanities.

Loma Linda University School of Medicine

Associate Dean for Admissions
Loma Linda University
School of Medicine
Loma Linda, CA 92350 · Tel: (714) 824-4468

Application and Acceptance (1987–88):
AMCAS application filing: June 15–Nov. 1, 1986
Fee: $35
Notification: Dec. 15, 1986–Aug. 1, 1987
Deposit: $100
Estimated new entrants: 140
School starts: July 1987

Approximate Expenses per Year (1985–86):
Tuition: $13,000
Fees: $500
Other costs: $5,000

Statistics (1985–86):
Applicants: 2,362 (1,146 in-state; 1,216 out-of-state)
New entrants: 141 (72 in-state; 69 out-of-state)
Mean GPA: 3.6

Requirements: MCAT, three years of college (bachelor's degree recommended), preference given to Seventh-Day Adventist Church members.

Required College Courses:	Years
General biology or zoology	1
General or inorganic chemistry	1
Organic chemistry	1
Physics	1
English (bachelor's degree requirement equivalency)	

Strongly recommended: clinical experience prior to affiliation.

University of Southern California School of Medicine

Office of Admissions
University of Southern California
School of Medicine
2025 Zonal Avenue
Los Angeles, CA 90033   Tel: (213) 224-7021

Application and Acceptance (1987–88):
AMCAS application filing: June 15–Nov. 1, 1986
Fee: $25
Offers Early Decision Plan
    EDP application filing: June 15–Aug. 1, 1986
    Notification by: Oct. 1, 1986
Regular applicants notified from: Oct. 15, 1986
Deposit: $100
Estimated new entrants: 136
School starts: Sept. 1987

Approximate Expenses per Year (1985–86):
Tuition: $14,600
Fees: $200
Other costs: $9,200

Statistics (1985–86):
Applicants: 3,790 (2,544 in-state; 1,246 out-of-state)
New entrants: 136 (117 in-state; 19 out-of-state)
Mean GPA: 3.52
Sex: 30% women; 70% men

Requirements: MCAT, three years of college (90 sem. hrs.),
    bachelor's degree preferred.

Required College Courses: Sem./Qtr.
Biology (with lab) 2/3
Inorganic chemistry (with lab) 2/3
Organic chemistry (with lab) 2/3
General physics (with lab) 2/3
English
Humanities

Recommended College Courses: Biochemistry.

Stanford University School of Medicine

Office of Admissions, Room 154
Stanford University
School of Medicine
851 Welch Road
Palo Alto, CA 94304-1677   Tel: (415) 497-6861

Application and Acceptance (1987–88):
AMCAS application filing: June 15–Oct. 15, 1986
Fee: $55
Offers Early Decision Plan
    EDP application filing: June 15–Aug. 1, 1986
    Notification by: Oct. 1, 1986
Regular applicants notified from: Oct. 15, 1986
Estimated new entrants: 86
School starts: Sept. 1987

Approximate Expenses per Year (1985–86):
Tuition: $10,600 (3-quarter academic year)
Other costs: $6,000

Statistics (1985–86):
Applicants: 5,518 (2,113 in-state; 3,405 out-of-state)
New entrants: 86 (34 in-state; 52 out-of-state)
Mean GPA: 3.6
Sex: 33% women; 67% men

Requirements: MCAT, bachelor's degree preferred.

Required College Courses: Years
Biological science (with lab) 1
Chemistry (with lab) 1
Organic chemistry (with lab) 1
Physics (with lab) 1

Recommended College Courses: Biochemistry, calculus, physical chemistry, behavioral sciences.

University of Colorado School of Medicine

Office of Admissions and Records
Box A054
University of Colorado
School of Medicine
4200 East Ninth Avenue
Denver, CO 80262   Tel: (303) 394-7676

Application and Acceptance (1987–88):
AMCAS application filing: June 15–Nov. 1, 1986
Fee: $20
Offers Early Decision Plan (residents and WICHE-certified
    applicants from Montana, Alaska, and Wyoming only)
    EDP application filing: June 15–Aug. 1, 1986
    Notification by: Oct. 1, 1986
Regular applicants notified: Oct. 15, 1986–March 15, 1987
Deposit: $200
Estimated new entrants: 125
School starts: Aug. 1987

Approximate Expenses per Year (1985–86):
Tuition: $6,400 (resident); $26,400 (nonresident)
Fees: $600
Other costs: $5,900

Statistics (1985–86):
Applicants: 830 (462 in-state; 368 out-of-state)
New entrants: 128 (126 in-state; 2 out-of-state)

Requirements: MCAT, bachelor's degree or 120 sem. hrs. college
    credit toward a degree major, preference given to Colorado
    residents and WICHE-certified residents of Western states.

Required College Courses: Sem. hrs.
General biology or zoology (with lab) 8
General chemistry (with lab) 8
Organic chemistry (with lab) 8
General physics (with lab) 8
Mathematics (incl. algebra and trigonometry or
    advanced-placement equivalent) 6
English literature or equivalent 6
English composition, creative writing, or equivalent 3

Recommended College Courses: Calculus, quantitative mathe-
    matically oriented physics.

University of Connecticut School of Medicine

Office of Admissions and Student Affairs
University of Connecticut
School of Medicine
University of Connecticut Health Center
263 Farmington Avenue
Farmington, CT 06032   Tel: (203) 674-2152

Application and Acceptance (1987–88):
AMCAS application filing: June 15–Dec. 1, 1986
Fee: $35
Offers Early Decision Plan
    EDP application filing: June 15–Aug. 1, 1986
    Notification by: Oct. 1, 1986
Regular applicants notified from: Oct. 15, 1986
Deposit: $100
Estimated new entrants: 88
School starts: Aug. 1987

Approximate Expenses per Year (1985–86):
Tuition: $3,600 (resident); $8,200 (nonresident)
Fees: $2,200
Other costs: $8,000

Statistics (1985–86):
Applicants: 1,554 (445 in-state; 1,109 out-of-state)
New entrants: 88 (85 in-state; 3 out-of-state)
Mean GPA: 3.5

Requirements: MCAT, three years of college (bachelor's degree recommended), preference given to Connecticut residents.

Required College Courses: Years
General biology or zoology (with lab)..1
General chemistry (with lab) 1
Organic chemistry (with lab) 1
General physics (with lab)..1

Yale University School of Medicine

Office of the Registrar
Yale University
School of Medicine
333 Cedar Street
New Haven, CT 06510   Tel: (203) 785-2643

Application and Acceptance (1987–88):
Application filing: June 1–Nov. 1, 1986
Fee: $50
Offers Early Decision Plan
    EDP application filing: June 1–Aug. 15, 1986
    Notification by: Oct. 1, 1986
Regular applicants notified: Dec. 15, 1986–April 15, 1987
Deposit: $100
Estimated new entrants: 102
School starts: Sept. 1987

Approximate Expenses per Year (1985–86):
Tuition: $11,800
Fees: $300
Other costs: $7,700

Statistics (1985–86):
Applicants: 2,919 (201 in-state; 2,718 out-of-state)
New entrants: 102 (8 in-state; 94 out-of-state)

Requirements: MCAT, four years of college study recommended.

Required College Courses: Years
General biology or zoology (with lab) 1
General or inorganic chemistry (with lab) 1
Organic chemistry (with lab) 1
General physics (with lab) 1

George Washington University
School of Medicine and Health Sciences

Office of Admissions
George Washington University
School of Medicine and Health Sciences
2300 Eye Street, N.W.
Washington, DC 20037   Tel: (202) 676-3506

Application and Acceptance (1987–88):
AMCAS application filing: June 15–Nov. 15, 1986
Fee: $40
Offers Early Decision Plan
    EDP application filing: June 15–Aug. 1, 1986
    Notification by: Oct. 1, 1986
Regular applicants notified: Oct. 15, 1986–Aug. 1987
Estimated new entrants: 150
School starts: Aug. 1987

Approximate Expenses per Year (1985–86):
Tuition: $18,800
Fees: $200
Other costs: $8,400

Statistics (1985–86):
Applicants: 6,352 (58 in-state; 6,294 out-of-state)
New entrants: 148 (6 in-state; 142 out-of-state)
Mean GPA: 3.4
Sex: 60% women; 40% men

Requirements: MCAT, three years of college (90 sem. hrs.),
    bachelor's degree preferred.

Required College Courses:	Sem. hrs.
Biology and/or zoology (with lab)	8
Inorganic chemistry (with lab)	8
Organic chemistry (with lab)	8
Physics (with lab)	8
English (composition and literature)	6

Georgetown University School of Medicine

Office of Admissions
Georgetown University
School of Medicine
3900 Reservoir Road, N.W.
Washington, DC 20007   Tel: (202) 625-7768

Application and Acceptance (1987–88):
AMCAS application filing: June 15–Nov. 15, 1986
Fee: $40
Offers Early Decision Plan
    EDP application filing: June 15–Aug. 1, 1986
    Notification by: Oct. 1, 1986
Regular applicants notified from: Oct. 15, 1986
Deposit: $100
Estimated new entrants: 205
School starts: Aug. 1987

Approximate Expenses per Year (1985–86):
Tuition: $20,600
Fees: $600
Other costs: $12,000

Statistics (1985–86):
Applicants: 6,916 (59 D.C.; 6,857 other)
New entrants: 205 (4 D.C.; 201 other)
Mean GPA: 3.4
Sex: 28.4% women; 71.6% men

Requirements: MCAT, three years of college (90 sem. hrs.),
    bachelor's degree highly desirable.

Required College Courses:	Sem./Qtr.
Biology (with lab)	2/3
Inorganic chemistry (with lab)	2/3
Organic chemistry (with lab)	2/3
General physics (with lab)	2/3
Mathematics	2/3
English	2/3

Howard University College of Medicine

Admissions Office
Howard University
College of Medicine
520 W Street, N.W.
Washington, DC 20059   Tel: (202) 636-6270

Application and Acceptance (1987–88):
AMCAS application filing: June 15–Dec. 15, 1986
Fee: $25
Notification from: Oct. 15, 1986
Deposit: $100
Estimated new entrants: 125
School starts: Aug. 1987

Approximate Expenses per Year (1985–86):
Tuition: $4,500
Fees: $400
Other costs: $8,900

Statistics (1985–86):
Applicants: 4,412 (91 D.C.; 4,321 other)
New entrants: 117 (12 D.C.; 105 other)
Sex: 46% women; 54% men

Requirements: MCAT, 62 hrs. of college credit.

Required College Courses:	Sem. hrs.
Biology or zoology	8
General chemistry	8
Organic chemistry	8
General physics	8
Mathematics	6
English	6

University of Florida College of Medicine

Chairman, Medical Selection Committee
Box J-216
J. Hillis Miller Health Center
University of Florida
College of Medicine
Gainesville, FL 32610   Tel: (904) 392-3071

Application and Acceptance (1987–88):
AMCAS application filing: June 15–Nov. 15, 1986
Fee: $15
Notification from: Oct. 15, 1986
Estimated new entrants: 85
School starts: Aug. 1987

Approximate Expenses per Year (1985–86):
Tuition and fees: $2,700 (resident); $6,100 (nonresident)
Other costs: $8,900

Statistics (1985–86):
Applicants: 1,553 (781 in-state; 772 out-of-state)
New entrants: 85 (82 in-state; 3 out-of-state)
Mean GPA: 3.6
Sex: 36% women; 64% men

Requirements: MCAT, bachelor's degree generally required, preference given to Florida residents.

Required College Courses: Sem. hrs.
Biology (with lab) 8
Inorganic chemistry (with lab) 8
Organic chemistry (with lab) 8
General physics (with lab) 8

Recommended College Courses: Liberal arts, humanities, and social, mathematical, biological, and behavioral sciences.

University of Miami School of Medicine

Office of Admissions
University of Miami
School of Medicine
P.O. Box 016159
Miami, FL 33101   Tel: (305) 547-6791

Application and Acceptance (1987–88):
Application filing: July 1–Dec. 15, 1986
Fee: $50
Notification from: Oct. 1986
Deposit: $50
Estimated new entrants: 138
School starts: Sept. 1987

Approximate Expenses per Year (1985–86):
Tuition: $10,500
Fees: $100
Other costs: $10,500

Statistics (1985–86):
Applicants: 907 (753 in-state; 154 out-of-state)
New entrants: 138 (133 in-state; 5 out-of-state)

Requirements: MCAT, 90 sem. hrs. of college credit.

Required College Courses: Sem.
General biology or zoology (incl. no more than 1 sem.
    botany) 2
Inorganic chemistry 2
Organic chemistry 2
General physics 2
Mathematics (incl. calculus) 1
English 2
Biochemistry or advanced chemistry ....(3 sem. hrs./4 qtr. hrs.)

Recommended College Courses: Humanities, arts, and social
    sciences.

University of South Florida College of Medicine

Admissions Office, Box 3
University of South Florida
College of Medicine
12901 North 30th Street
Tampa, FL 33612   Tel: (813) 974-2229

Application and Acceptance (1987–88):
Preliminary application filing (nonresident): July 1–Oct. 5, 1986
Formal application filing (resident): July 1–Dec. 1, 1986 (firm rule)
Fee: $15
Offers Early Decision Plan (residents only)
    EDP application filing: July 1–Aug. 1, 1986
    Notification by: Aug. 31, 1986
Regular applicants notified from: Aug. 31, 1986
Estimated new entrants: 96
School starts: Aug. 1987

Approximate Expenses per Year (1985–86):
Tuition: $2,800 (resident); $6,300 (nonresident)
Fees: $100
Other costs: $6,500

Statistics (1985–86):
Applicants: 931 (734 in-state; 197 out-of-state)
New entrants: 96 (95 in-state; 1 out-of-state)
Mean GPA: 3.6
Sex: 33% women; 67% men

Requirements: MCAT, three years of college (90 sem. hrs.),
    bachelor's degree recommended, preference given to Flori-
    da residents.

Required College Courses:	Sem.
General biology (with lab)	2
Mendelian genetics (lab optional)	1
General chemistry (with lab)	2
Organic chemistry (with lab)	2
General physics (with lab)	2
Mathematics	2
English	2
Statistics (mathematics or social science)	1

Recommended College Courses: Physical chemistry or biologi-
    cal chemistry, embryology, cell biology, comparative anatomy.

Emory University School of Medicine

Medical School Admissions, Room 303
Woodruff Health Sciences Center
Administration Building
Emory University
School of Medicine
Atlanta, GA 30322   Tel: (404) 727-5660

Application and Acceptance (1987–88):
AMCAS application filing: June 15–Oct. 15, 1986
Fee: $40
Notification: Oct. 15, 1986–March 15, 1987
Deposit: $50
Estimated new entrants: 110
School starts: Aug. 1987

Approximate Expenses per Year (1985–86):
Tuition: $11,200
Fees: $300
Other costs: $7,200

Statistics (1985–86):
Applicants: 3,751 (409 in-state; 3,342 out-of-state)
New entrants: 110 (57 in-state; 53 out-of-state)
Mean GPA: 3.59
Sex: 30% women; 70% men

Requirements: MCAT, three years of college (90 sem./135 qtr. hrs.).

Required College Courses: Years
Biology (with lab) 1
Inorganic chemistry (with lab) 1
Organic chemistry (with lab) ....(6 sem./10 qtr. hrs. min.)
Physics (with lab) 1
English...(6 sem./10 qtr. hrs. min.)
Humanities, behavioral science, social science....(18 sem./27 qtr. hrs. min.)

Recommended College Courses: Biochemistry.

Medical College of Georgia School of Medicine

Office of Student Affairs
Medical College of Georgia
School of Medicine
Augusta, GA 30912   Tel: (404) 828-3186

Application and Acceptance (1987–88):
AMCAS application filing: June 15–Dec. 1, 1986
Notification from: Oct. 15, 1986
Deposit: $50
Estimated new entrants: 180
School starts: Aug. 1987

Approximate Expenses per Year (1985–86):
Tuition: $2,400 (resident); $4,800 (nonresident)
Fees: $200
Other costs: $6,300

Statistics (1985–86):
Applicants: 1,021 (578 in-state; 443 out-of-state)
New entrants: 180 (178 in-state; 2 out-of-state)
Mean GPA: resident applicants, 3.45; GPA higher for nonresidents

Requirements: MCAT, three years of college (bachelor's degree recommended), preference given to Georgia residents.

Required College Courses: Years
Biology (with lab) 1
Inorganic chemistry (with lab) 1
Advanced chemistry (incl. 1 sem. or 2 qtrs. organic
    chemistry; lab) 1
Physics (incl. heat, light, sound, electricity, magnetism,
    mechanics; lab)
English (sufficient to satisfy bachelor's degree requirements)

Mercer University School of Medicine

Office of Admissions and Student Affairs
Mercer University
School of Medicine
Macon, GA 31207   Tel: (912) 744-2524

Application and Acceptance (1987–88):
AMCAS application filing: June 15–Dec. 1, 1986
Fee: $25
Offers Early Decision Plan
    EDP application filing: June 15–Aug. 1, 1986
    Notification by: Oct. 1, 1986
Regular applicants notified: Oct. 15, 1986–Aug. 18, 1987
Deposit: $100
Estimated new entrants: 48
School starts: Aug. 1987

Approximate Expenses per Year (1985–86):
Tuition: $11,500
Fees: $100
Other costs: $7,800

Statistics (1985–86):
Applicants: 858 (383 in-state; 475 out-of-state)
New entrants: 24 (24 in-state; 0 out-of-state)
Sex: 50% women; 50% men

Requirements: MCAT, three years of college (90 sem. hrs.).

Required College Courses: Years
Biology (with lab) 1
General or inorganic chemistry (with lab) 1
Organic chemistry or organic/biochemistry sequence (with lab) ...1
General physics (with lab)..1

Morehouse School of Medicine

Admissions and Student Affairs
Morehouse School of Medicine
720 Westview Drive, S.W.
Atlanta, GA 30310   Tel: (404) 752-1010

Application and Acceptance (1987–88):
AMCAS application filing: June 15–Dec. 1, 1986
Fee: $30
Offers Early Decision Plan (minority applicants only)
      EDP application filing: June 15–Aug. 1, 1986
      Notification by: Oct. 1, 1986
Regular applicants notified: Oct. 15, 1986–May 1, 1987
Deposit: $100
Estimated new entrants: 32
School starts: July 1987

Approximate Expenses per Year (1985–86):
Tuition: $9,500
Fees: $900
Other costs: $7,500

Statistics (1985–86):
Applicants: 1,846 (329 in-state; 1,517 out-of-state)
New entrants: 32 (20 in-state; 12 out-of-state)

Requirements: MCAT, 90 sem. or 135 qtr. hrs. of college credit,
    preference given to qualified residents of Alabama, Geor-
    gia, and New York.

Required College Courses: Sem./Qtr. hrs.
Biology (with lab) 8/12
General (inorganic) chemistry (with lab) 8/12
Organic chemistry (with lab) 8/12
Physics (with lab) 8/12
College mathematics..6/10
English (incl. composition) 6/10

Recommended College Courses: Biochemistry, embryology,
    genetics.

University of Hawaii
John A. Burns School of Medicine

Office of Student Affairs
University of Hawaii
John A. Burns School of Medicine
1960 East-West Road
Honolulu, Hawaii 96822   Tel: (808) 948-8300

Application and Acceptance (1987–88):
AMCAS application filing: June 15–Dec. 1, 1986
Offers Early Decision Plan (under which nonresidents must apply)
   EDP application filing: June 15–Aug. 1, 1986
   Notification by: Oct. 1, 1986
Regular applicants notified: Oct. 15, 1986–March 31, 1987
Estimated new entrants: 56
School starts: July 1987

Approximate Expenses per Year (1985–86):
Tuition: $3,100 (residents); $11,600 (nonresident)
Fees: $100
Other costs: $7,000

Statistics (1985–86):
Applicants: 424 (196 in-state; 228 out-of-state)
New entrants: 57 (54 in-state; 3 out-of-state)

Requirements: MCAT, three years of college (90 credits).

Required College Courses:	Sem. hrs.
Biology (incl. comparative anatomy)	10
General chemistry	4–8
Organic chemistry	8
Physics	8
Mathematics through precalculus	
English	
Humanities	

Recommended College Courses: Statistics, embryology, introductory genetics, foreign language, anthropology, physical chemistry, biochemistry, microbiology.

University of Chicago
Pritzker School of Medicine

Office of the Dean of Students
University of Chicago
Pritzker School of Medicine
Billings Hospital, Room P-130, Box 69
5841 South Maryland
Chicago, IL 60637   Tel: (312) 962-1937

Application and Acceptance (1987–88):
AMCAS application filing: June 15–Nov. 15, 1986
Fee: $35
Offers Early Decision Plan
    EDP application filing: June 15–Sept. 1, 1986
    Notification by: Oct. 1, 1986
Regular applicants notified: Nov. 1, 1986–April 15, 1987
Deposit: $50
Estimated new entrants: 104
School starts: Sept. 25, 1987

Approximate Expenses per Year (1985–86):
Tuition: $11,100
Fees: $500
Other costs: $7,100

Statistics (1985–86):
Applicants: 2,946 (615 in-state; 2,331 out-of-state)
New entrants: 104 (45 in-state; 59 out-of-state)
Average GPA: science, 3.71; nonscience, 3.7

Requirements: MCAT, three years of college (bachelor's degree
    preferred).

Required College Courses: Sem. hrs.
Biology (incl. 8 sem. hrs. with lab) 12
Chemistry (general/inorganic and organic, incl. aliphatic
    and aromatic compounds) 16
Physics (with lab) 8
English composition
Mathematics
Social sciences
Humanities

University of Health Sciences
Chicago Medical School

Office of Admissions
UHS/Chicago Medical School
3333 Green Bay Road
North Chicago, IL 60064   Tel: (312) 578-3206/3207

Application and Acceptance (1987–88):
AMCAS application filing: June 15–Nov. 15, 1986
Fee: $55
Offers Early Decision Plan
   EDP application filing: June 15–Aug. 1, 1986
   Notification by: Oct. 1, 1986
Regular applicants notified from: Nov. 15, 1986
Deposit: $100
Estimated new entrants: 150
School starts: July 1987

Approximate Expenses per Year (1985–86):
Tuition: $18,000
Fees: $600
Other costs: $8,300

Statistics (1985–86):
Applicants: 5,192 (868 in-state; 4,324 out-of-state)
New entrants: 150 (50 in-state; 100 out-of-state)
Mean GPA: 3.43

Requirements: MCAT, three years of college (135 qtr. hrs. min.), bachelor's degree preferred.

Required College Courses: Years
Biology or zoology (with lab) 1
Inorganic chemistry (with lab) 1
Organic chemistry (with lab) 1
General physics (with lab) 1

Recommended College Courses: Advanced sciences.

University of Illinois College of Medicine

Office of Admissions and Records
University of Illinois
College of Medicine
P.O. Box 6998
Chicago, IL 60680   Tel: (312) 996-7690

Application and Acceptance (1987–88):
AMCAS application filing: June 15–Dec. 1, 1986
Fee: $20
Offers Early Decision Plan
 EDP application filing: June 15–Aug. 1, 1986
 Notification by: Oct. 1, 1986
Regular applicants notified from: Oct. 15, 1986
Deposit: $100
Estimated new entrants: 331
School starts: Aug. 1987

Approximate Expenses per Year (1985–86):
Tuition: $3,800 (resident); $11,400 (nonresident)
Fees: $800
Other costs: $8,000

Statistics (1985–86):
Applicants: 3,018 (1,485 in-state; 1,533 out-of-state)
New entrants: 331 (300 in-state; 31 out-of-state)

Requirements: MCAT, bachelor's degree, preference given to Illinois residents.

Recommended College Courses: Biology, chemistry (incl. organic), physics or biophysics, behavioral science, mathematics (incl. calculus).

Loyola University of Chicago
Stritch School of Medicine

Director of Admissions
Loyola University of Chicago
Stritch School of Medicine
2160 South First Avenue
Maywood, IL 60153   Tel: (312) 531-3229

Application and Acceptance (1987–88):
AMCAS application filing: June 15–Nov. 15, 1986
Fee: $35
Offers Early Decision Plan
    EDP application filing: June 15–Aug. 1, 1986
    Notification by: Oct. 1, 1986
Regular applicants notified from: Oct. 15, 1986
Estimated new entrants: 130
School starts: Aug. 1987

Approximate Expenses per Year (1985–86):
Tuition: $12,000 (resident); $14,500 (nonresident)
Fees: $400
Other costs: $7,000

Statistics (1985–86):
Applicants: 5,387 (1,215 in-state; 4,172 out-of-state)
New entrants: 130 (71 in-state; 59 out-of-state)
Mean GPA: 3.46
Sex: 36% women; 64% men

Requirements: MCAT, bachelor's degree, preference given to Illinois residents.

Required College Courses: Years
Biology (with lab) 1
Inorganic chemistry (with lab) 1
Organic chemistry (may include sem. or qtr. of
    biochemistry; lab)...1
Physics (with lab) 1

Recommended College Courses: English, psychology, calculus, biochemistry, genetics.

Northwestern University Medical School

Northwestern University Medical School
303 East Chicago Avenue
Chicago, IL 60611   Tel: (312) 649-8206

Application and Acceptance (1987–88):
AMCAS application filing: June 15–Nov. 15, 1986
Fee: $45
Offers Early Decision Plan
    EDP application filing: June 15–Aug. 1, 1986
    Notification by: Oct. 1, 1986
Regular applicants notified from: Nov. 15, 1986
Estimated new entrants: 170
School starts: Sept. 1987

Approximate Expenses per Year (1985–86):
Tuition: $12,800
Fees: $200
Other costs: $6,300

Statistics (1985–86):
Applicants: 5,694 (1,014 in-state; 4,680 out-of-state)
New entrants: 170 (87 in-state; 83 out-of-state)
Mean GPA: 3.49
Sex: 33% women, 67% men

Requirements: MCAT, 135 qtr. hrs. or 90 sem. hrs. of college
    credit, bachelor's degree preferred.

Required College Courses:	Years
Biology	1
General chemistry	1
Organic chemistry	1
General physics	1
English	1

Rush Medical College of Rush University

Office of Admissions
524 Academic Facility
Rush Medical College of Rush University
600 South Paulina Street
Chicago, IL 60612   Tel: (312) 942-6913

Application and Acceptance (1987–88):
AMCAS application filing: June 15–Nov. 15, 1986
Fee: $25
Offers Early Decision Plan
    EDP application filing: June 15–Aug. 1, 1986
    Notification by: Oct. 1, 1986
Regular applicants notified from: Oct. 15, 1986
Deposit: $100
Estimated new entrants: 120
School starts: Sept. 1987

Approximate Expenses per Year (1985–86):
Tuition: $13,200
Fees: $300
Other costs: $8,800

Statistics (1985–86):
Applicants: 2,681 (1,272 in-state; 1,409 out-of-state)
New entrants: 120 (104 in-state; 16 out-of-state)

Requirements: MCAT, 90 sem. hrs. of college credit, preference given to Illinois residents.

Required College Courses: Sem.
Biology 2
Inorganic chemistry 2
Organic chemistry (may include 1 sem. of biochemistry) 2
General physics 2

Southern Illinois University School of Medicine

Office of Student Affairs
Southern Illinois University
School of Medicine
P.O. Box 3926
Springfield, IL 62708   Tel: (217) 782-2860

Application and Acceptance (1987–88):
AMCAS application filing: June 15–Nov. 15, 1986
Offers Early Decision Plan (residents only)
    EDP application filing: June 15–Aug. 1, 1986
    Notification by: Oct. 1, 1986
Regular applicants notified: Oct. 15, 1986–March 15, 1987
Deposit: $100
Estimated new entrants: 72
School starts: Aug. 1987

Approximate Expenses per Year (1985–86):
Tuition: $4,000 (resident); $12,000 (nonresident)
Fees: $700
Other costs: $7,700

Statistics (1985–86):
Applicants: 1,022 (920 in-state; 102 out-of-state)
New entrants: 72 (72 in-state; 0 out-of-state)
Mean GPA: 3.38
Sex: 32% women; 68% men

Requirements: MCAT, 90 sem. hrs. of college credit; preference given to Illinois residents who intend to practice
medicine in Illinois.

Recommended College Courses: General and organic chemistry
(2 yrs.), physics (1 yr.), biological or life sciences (1 yr.),
mathematics (incl. statistics), English composition (1 yr.).

Indiana University School of Medicine

Medical School Admissions Office
Fesler Hall 213
Indiana University
School of Medicine
1120 South Drive
Indianapolis, IN 46223   Tel: (317) 264-3772

Application and Acceptance (1987–88):
AMCAS application filing: June 15–Dec. 15, 1986
Fee: $20
Notification: Nov. 15, 1986–May 15, 1987
Estimated new entrants: 290
School starts: Aug. 1987

Approximate Expenses per Year (1985–86):
Tuition: $3,300 (resident); $7,700 (nonresident)
Other costs: $7,200

Statistics (1985–86):
Applicants: 1,366 (626 in-state; 740 out-of-state)
New entrants: 290 (282 in-state; 8 out-of-state)
Average GPA: 3.65
Sex: 31% women; 69% men

Requirements: MCAT, three years of college (90 sem. hrs.), bachelor's degree strongly recommended, preference given to Indiana residents.

Required College Courses: Years
Biology (with labs) 1
General chemistry (with labs) ....:...............1
Organic chemistry (with labs) 1
Physics (with labs) 1

University of Iowa College of Medicine

Coordinator of Admissions
101 College of Medicine Administration Building
University of Iowa
College of Medicine
Iowa City, IA 52242   Tel: (319) 353-6617

Application and Acceptance (1987–88):
AMCAS application filing: June 15–Dec. 1, 1986
Fee: $10
Offers Early Decision Plan (under which most nonresidents must apply)
    EDP application filing: June 15–Aug. 1, 1986
    Notification by: Oct. 1, 1986
Regular applicants notified: Dec. 15, 1986–Aug. 1987
Deposit: $50
Estimated new entrants: 175
School starts: Aug. 1987

Approximate Expenses per Year (1985–86):
Tuition: $3,500 (resident); $6,900 (nonresident)
Other costs: $5,600

Statistics (1985–86):
Applicants: 942 (343 in-state; 599 out-of-state)
New entrants: 175 (143 in-state; 32 out-of-state)
Average GPA: 3.6

Requirements: MCAT, 94 sem. hrs. of college credit (bachelor's degree recommended), preference given to Iowa residents.

Required College Courses:
Biological sciences (incl. animal biology, zoology and botany, advanced biology; lab)
Chemistry (general and organic; lab)
Physics (with lab)
Mathematics (incl. algebra, trigonometry, advanced mathematics)

Recommended College Courses: Rhetoric, literature, social and behavioral science, historical culture.

University of Kansas
College of Health Sciences and Hospital
School of Medicine

Director, Student Admissions and Records
University of Kansas
College of Health Sciences
39th and Rainbow Boulevard
Kansas City, KS 66103   Tel: (913) 588-7055

Application and Acceptance (1987–88):
AMCAS application filing: June 15–Nov. 1, 1986
Fee: $15 (nonresidents)
Offers Early Decision Plan (residents only)
    EDP application filing: June 15–Aug. 1, 1986
    Notification by: Oct. 1, 1986
Regular applicants notified from: Jan. 31, 1987
Deposit: $50
Estimated new entrants: 200
School starts: Aug. 1987

Approximate Expenses per Year (1985–86):
Tuition: $5,300 (resident); $10,500 (nonresident)
Fee: $200
Other costs: $7,000

Statistics (1985–86):
Applicants: 843 (311 in-state; 532 out-of-state)
New entrants: 192 (167 in-state; 25 out-of-state)
Mean GPA: 3.6

Requirements: MCAT, bachelor's degree preferred, preference given to residents of Kansas.

Required College Courses: Years
Biological science (incl. general biology, vertebrate
    zoology; lab) 1
Inorganic chemistry (with lab) 1
Organic chemistry (incl. aliphatic and aromatic
    compounds; lab) 1
Quantitative analytical chemistry ....(1 sem.)
Physics (mathematics based; lab) 1
Mathematics (differential and integral calculus) 1
English (bachelor's degree requirement equivalency) 1

Recommended College Courses: Statistics.

University of Kentucky College of Medicine

Admissions, Room MN-109A
University of Kentucky
College of Medicine
Albert B. Chandler Medical Center
800 Rose Street
Lexington, KY 40536-0084   Tel: (606) 233-6161

Application and Acceptance (1987–88):
AMCAS application filing: June 15–Nov. 15, 1986
Offers Early Decision Plan
    EDP application filing: June 15–Aug. 1, 1986
    Notification by: Oct. 1, 1986
Regular applicants notified from: Oct. 1, 1986
Deposit: $100
Estimated new entrants: 85
School starts: Aug. 1987

Approximate Expenses per Year (1985–86):
Tuition: $3,500 (resident); $9,400 (nonresident)
Fees: $200
Other costs: $7,500

Statistics (1985–86):
Applicants: 982 (405 in-state; 577 out-of-state)
New entrants: 95 (86 in-state; 9 out-of-state)
Mean GPA: 3.59
Sex: 32% women; 68% men

Requirements: MCAT, three years of college, preference given
    to Kentucky residents.

Required College Courses: Sem.
Biological sciences (with lab) 2
Chemistry (incl. inorganic and organic; lab) 4
Physics (with lab) 2
English (communication skills) 2

Recommended College Courses: Social sciences, humanities.

University of Louisville School of Medicine

Associate Dean for Admissions
University of Louisville
Health Sciences Center
School of Medicine
Louisville, KY 40292   Tel: (502) 588-5193

Application and Acceptance (1987–88):
AMCAS application filing: June 15–Nov. 15, 1986
Fee: $15
Offers Early Decision Plan
    EDP application filing: June 15–Aug. 1, 1986
    Notification by: Oct. 1, 1986
Regular applicants notified: Oct. 1, 1986–May 1, 1987
Deposit: $100
Estimated new entrants: 124
School starts: Aug. 1987

Approximate Expenses per Year (1985–86):
Tuition: $3,700 (resident); $9,000 (nonresident)
Fees: $200
Other costs: $7,500

Statistics (1985–86):
Applicants: 859 (425 in-state; 434 out-of-state)
New entrants: 124 (113 in-state; 11 out-of-state)
Mean GPA: 3.53
Sex: 36% women; 64% men

Requirements: MCAT, three years of college (90 sem. hrs.), bachelor's degree recommended; preference given to Kentucky residents.

Required College Courses:	Sem.
General biology (with lab)	2
Inorganic chemistry (with lab)	2
Organic chemistry (with lab)	2
General physics (with lab)	2
Mathematics (1 sem. calculus or 2 sem. other college math)	2
English	2

Recommended College Courses: Calculus.

Louisiana State University
School of Medicine in New Orleans

Admissions Office
Louisiana State University
School of Medicine in New Orleans
1542 Tulane Avenue
New Orleans, LA 70112-2822   Tel: (504) 568-6262

Application and Acceptance (1987–88):
AMCAS application filing: June 15–Nov. 15, 1986
Fee: $20 (residents only)
Notification: Nov. 15, 1986–Aug. 15, 1987
Estimated new entrants: 175
School starts: Aug. 1987

Approximate Expenses per Year (1985–86):
Tuition: $2,700
Fees: $200
Other costs: $8,500

Statistics (1985–86):
Applicants: 806 (631 in-state; 175 out-of-state)
New entrants: 175 (175 in-state; 0 out-of-state)
Mean GPA: 3.4
Sex: 33% women; 67% men

Requirements: MCAT, bachelor's degree strongly recommended; preference given to Louisiana residents.

Required College Courses: Sem. hrs./Qtr.
Biology (general zoology, embryology, comparative
    vertebrate anatomy; lab) 8
General or inorganic chemistry (with lab) 6
Organic chemistry (with lab) 6/8
Advanced chemistry (quantitative analysis, biochemistry,
    physical chemistry; lab) 3/4
Physics (incl. heat, light, sound, mechanics, electricity,
    magnetism; lab) 8
English 9

Recommended College Courses: Advanced mathematics, genetics, statistical methods, psychology, economics, history, social studies.

Louisiana State University
School of Medicine in Shreveport

Office of Student Admissions
Louisiana State University
School of Medicine in Shreveport
P.O. Box 33932
Shreveport, LA 71130-3932   Tel: (318) 674-5190

Application and Acceptance (1987–88):
AMCAS application filing: June 15–Nov. 15, 1986
Fee: $20
Notification from: Nov. 15, 1986
Deposit: $50
Estimated new entrants: 100
School starts: Aug. 1987

Approximate Expenses per Year (1985–86):
Tuition and fees: $2,200 (resident); $5,700 (nonresident)
Other costs: $7,200

Statistics (1985–86):
Applicants: 679 (548 in-state; 131 out-of-state)
New entrants: 100 (100 in-state; 0 out-of-state)
Mean GPA: 3.62
Sex: 20% women; 80% men

Requirements: MCAT, three years of college (90 sem. hrs.),
    bachelor's degree recommended; preference given to Loui-
    siana residents.

Required College Courses:	Sem. hrs.
Biology or zoology (with lab)	8
Inorganic chemistry (with lab)	6
Organic chemistry (with lab)	6
General physics (with lab)	8
English	9
Classic or modern language	6

Tulane University School of Medicine

Director of Admissions
Tulane University
School of Medicine
1430 Tulane Avenue
New Orleans, LA 70112   Tel: (504) 588-5187

Application and Acceptance (1987–88):
AMCAS application filing: June 15–Dec. 15, 1986
Fee: $55
Notification from: Oct. 15, 1986
Deposit: $100
Estimated new entrants: 148
School starts: Aug. 1987

Approximate Expenses per Year (1985–86):
Tuition: $9,300 (resident); $14,100 (nonresident)
Fees: $600
Other costs: $8,500

Statistics (1985–86):
Applicants: 6,741 (510 in-state; 6,231 out-of-state)
New entrants: 148 (38 in-state; 110 out-of-state)
Mean GPA: 3.5 (est.)

Requirements: MCAT, three years of college (90 sem. hrs.), bachelor's degree recommended.

Required College Courses:	Sem./Qtr.
Biology or zoology (with lab)	2/3
Inorganic chemistry (with lab)	2/3
Organic chemistry (with lab)	2/3
General physics (with lab)	2/3
English	(1 yr.)

Johns Hopkins University School of Medicine

Committee on Admissions
The Johns Hopkins University
School of Medicine
720 Rutland Avenue
Baltimore, MD 21205   Tel: (301) 955-3182

Application and Acceptance (1987–88):
Application filing: June 15–Nov. 1, 1986; *Jan. 31, 1987**
Fee: $50
Offers Early Decision Plan
    EDP application filing: June 15–Aug. 15, 1986
    Notification by: Oct. 1, 1986
Regular applicants notified: Nov. 15, 1986 (*June 15, 1987*)*–
    March 30, 1987 (*June 15, 1987*)*
Estimated new entrants: 120
School starts: Sept. 1987

Approximate Expenses per Year (1985–86):
Tuition: $10,300
Fees: $1,800
Other costs: $8,300

Statistics (1985–86):
Applicants: 2,487 (180 in-state; 2,307 out-of-state)
New entrants: 120 (21 in-state; 99 out-of-state)

Requirements: Bachelor's degree.

Required College Courses:	Sem. hrs.
General biology or zoology (with lab)	8
General chemistry (with lab)	8
Organic chemistry (with lab)	8
General physics (with lab)	8
Humanities, social and behavioral sciences	24
Calculus	4

* Dates in italics for juniors in FlexMed program.

University of Maryland School of Medicine

Dr. Ellen G. McDaniel
Committee on Admissions
Room 14-015
University of Maryland
School of Medicine
655 West Baltimore Street
Baltimore, MD 21201   Tel: (301) 528-7478/7479

Application and Acceptance (1987–88):
AMCAS application filing: June 15–Dec. 1, 1986
Fee: $20
Offers Early Decision Plan (residents and nonresidents)
    EDP application filing: June 15–Aug. 1, 1986
    Notification by: Oct. 1, 1986
Regular applicants notified: Oct. 15, 1986 through third day of
    classes
Deposit: $100 (nonrefundable)
Estimated new entrants: 150
School starts: Aug. 1987

Approximate Expenses per Year (1985–86):
Tuition: $4,900 (resident); $9,700 (nonresident)
Fees: $600
Other costs: $6,500

Statistics (1985–86):
Applicants: 1,692 (740 in-state; 952 out-of-state)
New entrants: 152 (134 in-state; 18 out-of-state)
Average GPA: 3.58
Sex: 34% women; 66% men

Requirements: MCAT, 90 sem. hrs. of college credit, bachelor's
    degree recommended, preference given to Maryland
    residents.

Required College Courses: Sem. hrs.
General biology or biological sciences 8
Inorganic chemistry 8
Organic chemistry 6
General physics 8
English 6

Uniformed Services University of the Health Sciences
F. Edward Hébert School of Medicine

Admissions Office, Room A-1041
Uniformed Services University
 of the Health Sciences
F. Edward Hébert School of Medicine
4301 Jones Bridge Road
Bethesda, MD 20814-4799   Tel: (301) 295-3101

Application and Acceptance (1987–88):
AMCAS application filing: June 15–Nov. 1, 1986
Notification from: Oct. 15, 1986
Estimated new entrants: 156
School starts: July 1987

Approximate Expenses per Year:
There are no tuition charges for attending the School of Medi-
    cine. Books, equipment, and instruments are also furnished
    without charge.

Statistics (1985–86):
Applicants: 3,965
New entrants: 157
Mean GPA: 3.54
Sex: 18% women; 82% men

Requirements: MCAT, bachelor's degree, U.S. citizen who will
    not be more than 32 years old as of 30 June in the year of
    contemplated graduation (may be waived), meeting the
    physical and personal qualifications for a commission in the
    uniformed services.

Required College Courses:	Sem.
General biology	8
General or inorganic chemistry	8
Organic chemistry	8
Physics	8
Mathematics (through calculus)	6
English	6

Boston University School of Medicine

Admissions Office
Boston University
School of Medicine
80 East Concord Street
Boston, MA 02118   Tel: (617) 247-6005

Application and Acceptance (1987–88):
AMCAS application filing: June 15–Nov. 1, 1986
Fee: $50
Offers Early Decision Plan
    EDP application filing: June 15–Aug. 1, 1986
    Notification by: Oct. 1, 1986
Regular applicants notified from: Nov. 1986
Estimated new entrants: 135
School starts: Aug. 1987

Approximate Expenses per Year (1985–86):
Tuition: $17,200
Fees: $1,500
Other costs: $10,000

Statistics (1985–86):
Applicants: 6,975 (981 in-state; 5,994 out-of-state)
New entrants: 135 (37 in-state; 98 out-of-state)

Requirements: MCAT, bachelor's degree.

Required College Courses: Years
Biology (with lab) 1
Inorganic chemistry (with lab) 1
Organic chemistry (with lab) 1
Physics (with lab) 1
Humanities 1
English (composition or literature) 1

Recommended College Courses: Quantitative chemistry, calculus.

Harvard Medical School

Director of Admissions
Harvard Medical School
25 Shattuck Street
Boston, MA 02115   Tel: (617) 732-1550

Application and Acceptance (1987–88):
Request for application until: Oct. 1, 1986   Fee: $50
Application filing: May–Oct. 15, 1986
Notification by: late Feb. 1987
Estimated new entrants: 165
School starts: Sept. 1987

Approximate Expenses per Year (1985–86):
Tuition: $11,200   Fees: $800   Other costs: $7,100

Statistics (1985–86):
Applicants: 3,222 (269 in-state; 2,953 out-of-state)
New entrants: 165 (23 in-state; 142 out-of-state)

Requirements: MCAT, three years of college.

Required College Courses: Years
Biology (cellular and molecular biology, structure and
    function of living organisms; lab) 1
Chemistry (with lab) 2
        (full-year courses in inorganic and organic chemistry
        are traditional; options that adequately prepare for
        study of biochemistry and molecular biology also
        acceptable)
Physics 1
Calculus 1
        (a course in statistics and familiarity with computers desirable)
English or other nonscience courses that involve
    substantial experience in expository writing 1
Advanced placement credits may be used to satisfy the calculus
    requirement and one semester of the chemistry and physics
    requirements.

Recommended College Courses: At least 16 credit hours should
    be completed in nonscience areas including literature,
    languages, the arts, humanities, and the social and behavioral
    sciences. Honors courses and independent study are
    encouraged.

University of Massachusetts Medical School

Interim Dean for Admissions
University of Massachusetts Medical School
55 Lake Avenue, North
Worcester, MA 01605   Tel: (617) 856-2323

Application and Acceptance (1987–88):
AMCAS application filing: June 15–Nov. 1, 1986
Fee: $20
Offers Early Decision Plan (residents only)
    EDP application filing: June 15–Aug. 1, 1986
    Notification by: Oct. 1, 1986
Regular applicants notified from: Oct. 15, 1986
Estimated new entrants: 100
School starts: Sept. 1987

Approximate Expenses per Year (1985–86):
Learning contract available to Massachusetts residents only:

Tuition Total	Due Immediately	Future Obligation
$5,600	$2,000	$3,600

Fees: $200
Other costs: $7,600

Statistics (1985–86):
Applicants: 875 (875 in-state; 0 out-of-state)
New entrants: 100 (100 in-state; 0 out-of-state)
Mean science GPA: 3.5
Sex: 43% women; 57% men

Requirements: MCAT, three years of college (bachelor's degree recommended); must be resident of Massachusetts.

Required College Courses: Years
Biology (with lab) 1
Inorganic chemistry (with lab) 1
Organic chemistry (with lab) 1
Physics (with lab) 1
English 1

Recommended College Courses: Biochemistry, calculus, statistics, sociology, psychology.

Tufts University School of Medicine

Committee on Admissions
Tufts University
School of Medicine
136 Harrison Avenue
Boston, MA 02111   Tel: (617) 956-6571

Application and Acceptance (1987–88):
AMCAS application filing: June 15–Nov. 1, 1986
Fee: $50
Offers Early Decision Plan
    EDP application filing: June 15–Aug. 1, 1986
    Notification by: Oct. 1, 1986
Regular applicants notified from: Nov. 1, 1986
Deposit: $100
Estimated new entrants: 146
School starts: Sept. 1987

Approximate Expenses per Year (1985–86):
Tuition: $16,000
Fees: $700
Other costs: $9,000

Statistics (1985–86):
Applicants: 6,267 (767 in-state; 5,500 out-of-state)
New entrants: 146 (51 in-state; 95 out-of-state)

Requirements: MCAT, three years of college (bachelor's degree preferred).

Required College Courses:	Years
Biology (with lab)	1
Chemistry (inorganic and organic, incl. quantitative analysis; lab)	2
Physics (with lab)	1
English (fluency in speech and composition)	

Recommended College Courses: Classical genetics, biochemistry.

Michigan State University
College of Human Medicine

College of Human Medicine
Office of Admissions
B-106 Clinical Center
Michigan State University
East Lansing, MI 48824-1313   Tel: (517) 353-9620

Application and Acceptance (1987–88):
AMCAS application filing: June 15–Nov. 15, 1986
Fee: $20
Offers Early Decision Plan
    EDP application filing: June 15–Aug. 1, 1986
    Notification by: Oct. 1, 1986
Regular applicants notified from: Oct. 15, 1986
Deposit: $50
Estimated new entrants: 106
School starts: Sept. 1987

Approximate Expenses per Year (1985–86):
Tuition: $4,700 (resident); $9,600 (nonresident)
Other costs: $7,400

Statistics (1985–86):
Applicants: 2,203 (1,087 in-state; 1,116 out-of-state)
New entrants: 106 (86 in-state; 20 out-of-state)

Requirements: MCAT, three years of college (bachelor's degree highly recommended), preference given to Michigan residents.

Required College Courses: Sem./term credits
Biological sciences (incl. 3 sem. or 5 term credits lab) 6/9
Chemistry (incl. inorganic and organic; 3 sem. or 5 term
    credits lab) 8/12
Physics (incl. lab) 6/9
English (composition and literature) 6/9
Psychology and/or sociology 6/9
Nonscience areas (may incl. English and social sciences) ...18/27

University of Michigan Medical School

Admissions Office
M4303 Medical Science Building I
University of Michigan Medical School
1301 Catherine Road
Ann Arbor, MI 48109-0010   Tel: (313) 764-6317

Application and Acceptance (1987–88):
AMCAS application filing: June 15–Nov. 15, 1986
Fee: $20
Offers Early Decision Plan
     EDP application filing: June 15–Aug. 1, 1986
     Notification by: Oct. 1, 1986
Regular applicants notified from: Sept. 1, 1986
Deposit: $100
Estimated new entrants: 167
School starts: Aug. 1987

Approximate Expenses per Year (1985–86):
Tuition: $5,500 (resident); $10,400 (nonresident)
Fees: $100
Other costs: $5,400

Statistics (1985–86):
Applicants: 3,090 (1,049 in-state; 2,041 out-of-state)
New entrants: 167 (133 in-state; 34 out-of-state)

Requirements: MCAT, 90 sem. hrs. of college credit, prefer-
     ence given to Michigan residents.

Required College Courses: Sem. hrs.
Biology (with 3 hrs. lab) 6
Chemistry (general/inorganic and organic; lab) 8
Physics (with lab) 6
English (composition and literature) 6
Nonscience/humanities 18

Recommended College Courses: Advanced biology (especially
     zoology) and/or chemistry.

Wayne State University School of Medicine

Director of Admissions
Wayne State University
School of Medicine
540 East Canfield
Detroit, MI 48201   Tel: (313) 577-1466

Application and Acceptance (1987–88):
AMCAS application filing: June 15–Dec. 15, 1986
Fee: $25
Offers Early Decision Plan
    EDP application filing: June 15–Aug. 1, 1986
    Notification by: Oct. 1, 1986
Regular applicants notified from: Oct. 1, 1986
Deposit: $50
Estimated new entrants: 256
School starts: Aug. 1987

Approximate Expenses per Year (1985–86):
Tuition: $5,400 (resident); $10,700 (nonresident)
Fees: $200
Other costs: $8,000

Statistics (1985–86):
Applicants: 1,830 (1,231 in-state; 599 out-of-state)
New entrants: 250 (237 in-state; 13 out-of-state)
Mean GPA: 3.5

Requirements: MCAT, bachelor's degree generally required, preference given to Michigan residents.

Required College Courses: Years
General biology or zoology (with lab) 1
Genetics ....(1 course)
Inorganic chemistry (with lab) 1
Organic chemistry (with lab) 1
General physics (with lab) 1
English 1

Recommended College Courses: Psychology, social sciences.

Mayo Medical School

Admissions Committee
Mayo Medical School
200 First Street, S.W.
Rochester, MN 55905   Tel: (507) 284-2316

Application and Acceptance (1987–88):
AMCAS application filing: June 15–Dec. 15, 1986
Fee: $40
Offers Early Decision Plan
    EDP application filing: June 15–Aug. 1, 1986
    Notification by: Oct. 1, 1986
Regular applicants notified from: Oct. 15, 1986
Deposit: $100
Estimated new entrants: 40
School starts: Sept. 1987

Approximate Expenses per Year (1985–86):
Tuition and fees: $7,000 (resident); $14,900 (nonresident)
Other costs: $6,900

Statistics (1985–86):
Applicants: 1,271 (500 in-state; 771 out-of-state)
New entrants: 40 (20 in-state; 20 out-of-state)
Mean GPA: 3.57
Sex: 40% women; 60% men

Requirements: MCAT, bachelor's degree required.

Required College Courses:	Years
Biology and/or zoology	1
Chemistry (incl. organic)	2
Physics (with lab)	1

University of Minnesota, Duluth
School of Medicine

Office of Admissions, Room 107
University of Minnesota, Duluth
School of Medicine
2400 Oakland Avenue
Duluth, MN 55812   Tel: (218) 726-8511

Application and Acceptance (1987–88):
AMCAS application filing: June 15–Nov. 15, 1986
Offers Early Decision Plan
     EDP application filing: June 15–Aug. 1, 1986
         Notification by: Oct. 1, 1986
Regular applicants notified from: Oct. 15, 1986
Estimated new entrants: 48
School starts: Sept. 1987

Approximate Expenses per Year (1985–86):
Tuition: $6,100 (resident); $12,200 (nonresident)
Fees: $300
Other costs: $6,200

Statistics (1985–86):
Applicants: 596 (466 in-state; 130 out-of-state)
New entrants: 48 (48 in-state; 0 out-of-state)
Mean GPA: 3.4
Sex: 48% women; 52% men

Requirements: MCAT, bachelor's degree, preference given to
     residents of Minnesota.

Required College Courses: Years
General biology (with lab)..1
General physics (with lab)...1
Chemistry (incl. organic; lab) 2
English composition 1
Mathematics (incl. differential and integral
     calculus) ....(8 sem. hrs.)
Humanities (min. 1 upper-division course) ....(8 sem. hrs.)
Behavioral sciences (min. 1 upper-division course)
         ....(8 sem. hrs.)

University of Minnesota Medical School, Minneapolis

Associate Dean, Student Affairs and Admissions
Box 293, Mayo Memorial Building
University of Minnesota
Medical School, Minneapolis
420 Delaware Street, S.E.
Minneapolis, MN 55455   Tel: (612) 373-8091

Application and Acceptance (1987–88):
AMCAS application filing: June 15–Nov. 15, 1986
Offers Early Decision Plan (under which nonresidents must apply)
    EDP application filing: June 15–Aug. 1, 1986
    Notification by: Oct. 1, 1986
Regular applicants notified: Nov. 15, 1986–May 15, 1987
Estimated new entrants: 220
School starts: Sept. 1987

Approximate Expenses per Year (1985–86):
Tuition: $6,000 (resident); $12,000 (nonresident)
Fees: $400
Other costs: $5,600

Statistics (1985–86):
Applicants: 1,136 (745 in-state; 391 out-of-state)
New entrants: 238 (227 in-state; 11 out-of-state)
Mean GPA: 3.5
Sex: 40% women; 60% men

Requirements: MCAT, bachelor's degree, preference given to Minnesota residents.

Required College Courses: Qtr.
General biology or zoology 2
General or inorganic chemistry 2
Organic chemistry 2
Quantitative analysis 1
General physics 3
English ....(1 yr.)
Humanities, social sciences, other liberal arts ....(27 qtr. hrs.)
Calculus

Recommended College Courses: Genetics, psychology.

University of Mississippi School of Medicine

Division of Student Services and Records
University of Mississippi
School of Medicine
2500 North State Street
Jackson, MS 39216   Tel: (601) 987-4580

Application and Acceptance (1987–88):
AMCAS application filing: June 15–Dec. 1, 1986
Offers Early Decision Plan (residents only)
    EDP application filing: June 15–Aug. 1, 1986
    Notification by: Oct. 1, 1986
Regular applicants notified from: Oct. 15, 1986
Deposit: $50 (resident); $100 (nonresident)
Estimated new entrants: 110
School starts: Aug. 1987

Approximate Expenses per Year (1985–86):
Tuition: $5,000 (resident); $9,000 (nonresident)
Fees: $100
Other costs: $7,600

Statistics (1985–86):
Applicants: 495 (290 in-state; 205 out-of-state)
New entrants: 110 (110 in-state; 0 out-of-state)
Mean GPA: 3.5

Requirements: MCAT, three years of college (90 sem. hrs.), bachelor's degree recommended, preference given to Mississippi residents.

Required College Courses: Sem./Qtr.
General biology or zoology (with lab) 2/3
Inorganic or general chemistry (with lab) 2/3
Organic chemistry (with lab) 2/3
General physics (with lab) 2/3
Mathematics (min. 1 sem. each algebra and trigonometry;
    or 2 sem. analytical geometry and calculus)....................2/3
English composition 2/3
Advanced science (with lab) 2/3

Recommended College Courses: Well-rounded education including courses in the humanities.

University of Missouri, Columbia
School of Medicine

Associate Dean for Student Affairs
M222 Medical Sciences Building
University of Missouri, Columbia
School of Medicine
One Hospital Drive
Columbia, MO 65212   Tel: (314) 882-2923

Application and Acceptance (1987–88):
AMCAS application filing: June 15–Nov. 15, 1986
Offers Early Decision Plan
    EDP application filing: June 15–Aug. 1, 1986
    Notification by: Oct. 1, 1986
Regular applicants notified from: Oct. 1, 1986
Deposit: $100
Estimated new entrants: 110   School starts: Aug. 1987

Approximate Expenses per Year (1985–86):
Tuition: $5,300 (resident); $8,300 (nonresident)
Fees: $100   Other costs: $7,000

Statistics (1985–86):
Applicants: 865 (395 in-state; 470 out-of-state)
New entrants: 110 (103 in-state; 7 out-of-state)
Mean GPA: 3.44
Sex: 32% women; 68% men

Requirements: MCAT, 90 sem. hrs. of college credit (bachelor's degree strongly recommended), preference given to Missouri residents.

Required College Courses: Sem. hrs.
General biology (with lab)...8
Biology or zoology (may incl. comparative anatomy,
    embryology, genetics)...6
Inorganic chemistry (with lab) 8
Organic chemistry (with lab) 8
General physics (with lab)..8
Mathematics (algebra, calculus or calculus eligibility,
    statistics, trigonometry) ....(2 sem.)
English (composition)...(2 sem.)

Recommended College Courses: Social sciences, humanities.

University of Missouri, Kansas City
School of Medicine

University Admissions Office
University of Missouri, Kansas City
5100 Rockhill Road
Kansas City, MO 64110   Tel: (816) 932-4444

Application and Acceptance (1987–88):
Application filing: Sept. 1, 1986–Jan. 1, 1987
Fee: $50 (nonresident only)
Notification: March 1–May 1 (flexible), 1987
Deposit: $100
Estimated new entrants: 100
School starts: Aug. 1987

Approximate Expenses per Year (1985–86):
Tuition:

Resident:	$6,200 (yrs. 1 and 2)
	$7,100 (yrs. 3–6)
Nonresident:	$9,600 (yrs. 1 and 2)
	$11,100 (yrs. 3–6)

Other costs: $3,100

Statistics (1985–86):
Applicants: 510 (403 in-state; 107 out-of-state)
New entrants: 100 (82 in-state; 18 out-of-state)

Requirements: Six-year baccalaureate-medical program requires that student be graduated from high school, score 27 or higher on ACT, and demonstrate ability to perform successfully at college level. Applicants who have already begun college not eligible.

Required Courses (high school level):   Years
Mathematics 4
Physics 1
Chemistry 1
Biology 1
English 4

Saint Louis University School of Medicine

Ms. Nancy McPeters
Assistant to the Dean of Admissions
Saint Louis University
School of Medicine
1402 South Grand Boulevard
St. Louis, MO 63104   Tel: (314) 577-8205

Application and Acceptance (1987–88):
AMCAS application filing: June 15–Dec. 15, 1986
Fee: $45
Offers Early Decision Plan
    EDP application filing: June 15–Aug. 1, 1986
    Notification by: Oct. 1, 1986
Regular applicants notified from: Oct. 15, 1986
Deposit: $100
Estimated new entrants: 155
School starts: Sept. 1987

Approximate Expenses per Year (1985–86):
Tuition and fees: $14,500
Other costs: $7,000

Statistics (1985–86):
Applicants: 4,878 (301 in-state; 4,577 out-of-state)
New entrants: 158 (29 in-state; 129 out-of-state)
Mean GPA: 3.67
Sex: 21% women; 79% men

Requirements: MCAT, 90 sem. hrs. (135 qtr. hrs.) of college
    credit, bachelor's degree recommended.

Required College Courses: Sem. hrs.
General biology or zoology (with lab)..8
Inorganic chemistry (with lab) 8
Organic chemistry (with lab) 8
Physics (with lab) 8
English..6
Other humanities and behavioral sciences 12

Washington University School of Medicine

Admissions Office
Washington University
School of Medicine
660 South Euclid Avenue
St. Louis, MO 63110   Tel: (314) 362-6856

Application and Acceptance (1987–88):
AMCAS application filing: June 15–Nov. 1, 1986
Fee: $45
Offers Early Decision Plan
    EDP application filing: June 15–Aug. 1, 1986
    Notification by: Oct. 1, 1986
Regular applicants notified: Oct. 15, 1986–Aug. 21, 1987
Deposit: $100
Estimated new entrants: 120
School starts: Aug. 1987

Approximate Expenses per Year (1985–86):
Tuition: $13,700
Other costs: $7,300

Statistics (1985–86):
Applicants: 4,779 (215 in-state; 4,564 out-of-state)
New entrants: 130 (11 in-state; 119 out-of-state)
Mean GPA: 3.81
Sex: 27% women; 73% men

Requirements: MCAT, 90 sem. hrs. of college credit.

Required College Courses:	Years
Biological science	1
General or inorganic chemistry	1
Organic chemistry	1
Physics	1
Mathematics (incl. differential and integral calculus)	1

Recommended College Courses: Physical chemistry.

Creighton University School of Medicine

Health Sciences Admissions Office
Creighton University
School of Medicine
California at 24th Street
Omaha, NE 68178   Tel: (402) 280-2798

Application and Acceptance (1987–88):
AMCAS application filing: June 1–Dec. 15, 1986
Fee: $40
Offers Early Decision Plan
    EDP application filing: June 1–Aug. 1, 1986
    Notification by: Oct. 1, 1986
Regular applicants notified from: Jan. 15, 1987
Deposit: $100
Estimated new entrants: 110
School starts: Aug. 1987

Approximate Expenses per Year (1985–86):
Tuition: $10,900
Fees: $600
Other costs: $5,600

Statistics (1985–86):
Applicants: 5,772 (258 in-state; 5,514 out-of-state)
New entrants: 110 (28 in-state; 82 out-of-state)
Mean GPA: 3.46
Sex: 32% women; 68% men

Requirements: MCAT, three years of college (90 sem. hrs.),
bachelor's degree recommended, preference given to Mid-
western states residents and residents from states that do
not have medical schools.

Required College Courses:	Sem. hrs.
General biology (with lab)	8
Inorganic chemistry (with lab)	8
Organic chemistry (with lab)	8–10
General physics (with lab)	8
English	6

University of Nebraska College of Medicine

Chairman, Admissions Committee
Room 5017, Wittson Hall
University of Nebraska
College of Medicine
42nd Street and Dewey Avenue
Omaha, NE 68105   Tel: (402) 559-4205

Application and Acceptance (1987–88):
AMCAS application filing: June 15–Nov. 15, 1986
Notification: Dec. 19, 1986–May 1, 1987
Deposit: $100
Estimated new entrants: 120
School starts: Aug. 1987

Approximate Expenses per Year (1985–86):
Tuition: $3,200 (resident); $5,600 (nonresident)
Fees: $300
Other costs: $5,200

Statistics (1985–86):
Applicants: 1,087 (328 in-state; 759 out-of-state)
New entrants: 132 (123 in-state; 9 out-of-state)
Mean GPA: 3.48
Sex: 32% women; 68% men

Requirements: MCAT, three years of college (90 sem. hrs.),
bachelor's degree strongly recommended, preference given
to residents of Nebraska.

Required College Courses: Years
Biology (with lab) 1
Inorganic chemistry (with lab) 1
Organic chemistry (with lab) 1
Physics (with lab) 1
Humanities and/or social sciences (12–16 sem. hrs.) 2
Calculus or statistics
English (composition or writing)

University of Nevada School of Medicine

Office of Admissions
University of Nevada
School of Medicine
Reno, NV 89557   Tel: (702) 784-6001

Application and Acceptance (1987–88):
AMCAS application filing: June 15–Nov. 1, 1986
Fee: $35
Offers Early Decision Plan (residents only)
    EDP application filing: June 15–Aug. 1, 1986
    Notification by: Oct. 1, 1986
Regular applicants notified: Jan. 15–Summer, 1987
Estimated new entrants: 48
School starts: Aug. 1987

Approximate Expenses per Year (1985–86):
Tuition and fees: $4,200 (resident); $10,000 (nonresident)
Other costs: $8,000

Statistics (1985–86):
Applicants: 417 (141 in-state; 276 out-of-state)
New entrants: 48 (46 in-state; 2 out-of-state)
Mean GPA: 3.5
Sex: 27% women; 73% men

Requirements: MCAT, three years of college (90 sem. hrs.),
    bachelor's degree strongly recommended, preference given
    to Nevada residents.

Required College Courses: Sem. hrs.
Biology 16
Chemistry 8
Organic chemistry 8
Physics 8
Behavioral sciences (incl. 3 sem. hrs. upper-division
    credit) 9

Recommended College Courses: Calculus, biochemistry,
    genetics, embryology.

Dartmouth Medical School

Office of Admissions
    and Financial Aid
Dartmouth Medical School
Hanover, NH 03756   Tel: (603) 646-7505

Application and Acceptance (1987–88):
AMCAS application filing: June 15–Nov. 1, 1986
Fee: $55
Offers Early Decision Plan
    EDP application filing: June 15–Aug. 1, 1986
    Notification by: Sept. 1, 1986
Regular applicants notified: Nov. 15, 1986–May 1987
Estimated new entrants: 84
School starts: Sept. 1987

Approximate Expenses per Year (1985–86):
Tuition: $13,800
Fees: $200
Other costs: $7,000

Statistics (1985–86):
Applicants: 3,970 (64 in-state; 3,906 out-of-state)
New entrants: 86 (14 in-state; 72 out-of-state)

Requirements: MCAT.

Required College Courses:	Years
General biology	1
Inorganic chemistry	1
Organic chemistry	1
Physics	1
Calculus	½
English (written and oral proficiency)	

University of Medicine and Dentistry of New Jersey
New Jersey Medical School

Director of Admissions
UMDNJ–New Jersey Medical School
100 Bergen Street
Newark, NJ 07103   Tel: (201) 456-4631

Application and Acceptance (1987–88):
AMCAS application filing: June 15–Dec. 15, 1986
Fee: $25
Offers Early Decision Plan (exceptional residents only)
    EDP application filing: June 15–Aug. 1, 1986
    Notification by: Oct. 1, 1986
Regular applicants notified from: Nov. 1, 1986 (approx.)
Deposit: $100
Estimated new entrants: 170
School starts: Aug. 1987

Approximate Expenses per Year (1985–86):
Tuition: $7,200 (resident); $9,000 (nonresident)
Fees: $200
Other costs: $7,000

Statistics (1985–86):
Applicants: 2,391 (1,092 in-state; 1,299 out-of-state)
New entrants: 170 (162 in-state; 8 out-of-state)
Average GPA: 3.36
Sex: 35% women; 65% men

Requirements: MCAT, three years of college (90 credit hrs.), preference given to residents of New Jersey.

Required College Courses: Sem. hrs.
Biology (1 yr. each general and advanced biology,
    excl. of botany and invertebrate zoology; lab) 12
Organic chemistry (with lab) 8
Other chemistry (inorganic, physical, analytical,
    biochemistry; lab) 8
General physics (with lab) 8
English 6

Recommended College Courses: Mathematics.

University of Medicine and Dentistry of New Jersey
Rutgers Medical School

Office of Admissions
UMDNJ–Rutgers Medical School
P.O. Box 101
Piscataway, NJ 08854   Tel: (201) 463-4576

Application and Acceptance (1987–88):
AMCAS application filing: June 15–Dec. 15, 1986
Fee: $25
Offers Early Decision Plan
    EDP application filing: June 15–Aug. 1, 1986
    Notification by: Oct. 1, 1986
Regular applicants notified from: Oct. 15, 1986
Deposit: $50
Estimated new entrants: 130
School starts: Aug. 1987

Approximate Expenses per Year (1985–86):
Tuition: $7,200 (resident); $9,000 (nonresident)
Fees: $200
Other costs: $7,200

Statistics (1985–86):
Applicants: 2,630 (1,102 in-state; 1,528 out-of-state)
New entrants: 130 (119 in-state; 11 out-of-state)
Mean GPA: 3.43
Sex: 40% women; 60% men

Requirements: MCAT, three years of college (90 sem. hrs.), preference given to New Jersey residents.

Required College Courses: Years
Biology (with lab) 1
Inorganic chemistry (with lab) 1
Organic chemistry (with lab) 1
Physics (with lab) 1
Mathematics ....(1 sem.)
English...1

Recommended College Courses: Humanities, behavioral sciences.

University of New Mexico School of Medicine

Office of Admissions, Room 114
Basic Medical Sciences Building
University of New Mexico
School of Medicine
Albuquerque, NM 87131   Tel: (505) 277-4766

Application and Acceptance (1987–88):
AMCAS application filing: June 15–Dec. 1, 1986
Fee: $10
Offers Early Decision Plan (under which nonresidents must apply)
    EDP application filing: June 15–Aug. 1, 1986
    Notification by: Oct. 1, 1986
Regular applicants notified: Nov. 15, 1986–March 15, 1987
Estimated new entrants: 73
School starts: Aug. 1987

Approximate Expenses per Year (1985–86):
Tuition: $1,200 (resident); $3,300 (nonresident)
Fees: $100
Other costs: $7,800

Statistics (1985–86):
Applicants: 416 (217 in-state; 199 out-of-state)
New entrants: 73 (69 in-state; 4 out-of-state)
Average GPA: 3.4
Sex: 41% women; 59% men

Requirements: MCAT, three years of college (bachelor's degree recommended), preference given to residents of New Mexico and WICHE-certified residents of Western states.

Required College Courses:	Sem. hrs.
General biology or zoology (with lab)	8
General or inorganic chemistry (with lab)	8
Organic chemistry (with lab)	8
General physics	6
Mathematics	6

Recommended College Courses: Biochemistry, calculus, Spanish.

Albany Medical College of Union University

Director of Admissions
Albany Medical College
   of Union University
47 New Scotland Avenue
Albany, NY 12208   Tel: (518) 445-5521

Application and Acceptance (1987–88):
Application filing: July 1–Nov. 1, 1986
Fee: $60
Notification from: Oct. 15, 1986
Deposit: $100
Estimated new entrants: 128
School starts: Aug. 1987

Approximate Expenses per Year (1985–86):
Tuition: $17,000
Other costs: $7,200

Statistics (1985–86):
Applicants: 2,682 (1,715 in-state; 967 out-of-state)
New entrants: 127 (96 in-state; 31 out-of-state)
Mean GPA: 3.3

Requirements: MCAT, minimum of three years of college (bachelor's degree recommended).

Required College Courses: Sem. hrs./Qtr. hrs.
Biology or zoology (excl. of botany; lab) 6/9
Inorganic chemistry (with lab)...6/9
Organic chemistry (with lab) 6/9
General physics (incl. mechanics, heat, light,
    sound, electricity; lab) 6/9
English (facility in writing and speaking)

Albert Einstein College of Medicine of Yeshiva University

Admissions Officer
Albert Einstein College of Medicine
   of Yeshiva University
1300 Morris Park Avenue
Bronx, NY 10461   Tel: (212) 430-2106

Application and Acceptance (1987–88):
AMCAS application filing: June 15–Nov. 15, 1986
Fee: $55
Notification from: Jan. 15, 1987
Deposit: $100
Estimated new entrants: 179
School starts: Aug. 1987

Approximate Expenses per Year (1985–86):
Tuition: $13,100
Fees: $400
Other costs: $6,800

Statistics (1985–86):
Applicants: 5,525 (2,324 in-state; 3,201 out-of-state)
New entrants: 176 (126 in-state; 50 out-of-state)
Mean GPA: applicants for admission, 3.57; accepted students
   significantly higher
Sex: 40% women; 60% men

Requirements: MCAT, three years of college (bachelor's degree
   preferred).

Required College Courses: Years
Biology (with lab) 1
General chemistry (with lab) 1
Organic chemistry (with lab) 1
Physics (with lab) 1
Mathematics 1
English...1

Recommended College Courses: Quantitative analysis, biochemistry, physical chemistry, calculus, genetics.

Columbia University College of Physicians and Surgeons

Admissions Office
Columbia University
College of Physicians and Surgeons
630 West 168th Street
New York, NY 10032   Tel: (212) 694-3595/3596

Application and Acceptance (1987–88):
Application filing: June 1–Oct. 15, 1986
Fee: $50
Notification from: Feb. 1, 1987
Estimated new entrants: 148
School starts: Sept. 1987

Approximate Expenses per Year (1985–86):
Tuition: $13,100
Fees: $2,200
Other costs: $6,500

Statistics (1985–86):
Applicants: 3,125
New entrants: 148 (74 in-state; 74 out-of-state)

Requirements: MCAT, three years of college (bachelor's degree recommended).

Required College Courses: Years
Biology (mammalian preferred) 1
General chemistry 1
Organic chemistry 1
Physics 1
English 1

Cornell University Medical College

Office of Admissions
Cornell University Medical College
445 East 69th Street
New York, NY 10021   Tel: (212) 472-5673

Application and Acceptance (1987–88):
AMCAS application filing: June 15–Nov. 15, 1986
Fee: $45
Notification from: Oct. 15, 1986
Deposit: $100
Estimated new entrants: 101
School starts: Aug. 1987

Approximate Expenses per Year (1985–86):
Tuition: $14,600
Other costs: $7,000

Statistics (1985–86):
Applicants: 5,445 (1,854 in-state; 3,591 out-of-state)
New entrants: 101 (51 in-state; 50 out-of-state)
Mean science GPA: 3.56
Sex: 38% women; 62% men

Requirements: MCAT, three years of college (bachelor's degree
   recommended).

Required College Courses:	Sem. hrs.
General biology or zoology	6
General chemistry	6
Organic chemistry	6
General physics	6
English	6

Recommended College Courses: Calculus.

Mount Sinai School of Medicine
of the City University of New York

Jay A. Cohen
Assistant Dean, Admissions and Student Affairs
Room 5-04, Annenberg Building
Mount Sinai School of Medicine
One Gustave L. Levy Place
New York, NY 10029   Tel: (212) 650-6696

Application and Acceptance (1987–88):
Application filing: Aug. 1–Oct. 31, 1986
Fee: $75
Notification from: Nov. 1, 1986
Deposit: $100
Estimated new entrants: 100
School starts: Aug. 1987

Approximate Expenses per Year (1985–86):
Tuition: $14,000
Fees: $500
Other costs: $7,800

Statistics (1985–86):
Applicants: 2,797 (1,699 in-state; 1,098 out-of-state)
New entrants: 105 (78 in-state; 27 out-of-state)
Mean GPA: 3.6
Sex: 39% women; 61% men

Requirements: MCAT, three years of college (bachelor's degree
recommended).

Required College Courses:	Years
Biology	1
Inorganic chemistry	1
Organic chemistry	1
Physics	1
Mathematics	1
English	1

New York Medical College

Office of Admissions
Room 338, Elmwood Hall
New York Medical College
Valhalla, NY 10595   Tel: (914) 993-4507

Application and Acceptance (1987–88):
AMCAS application filing: June 15–Dec. 1, 1986
Fee: $50
Offers Early Decision Plan
    EDP application filing: June 15–Aug. 1, 1986
    Notification by: Oct. 1, 1986
Regular applicants notified: Jan. 15–Aug. 1987
Deposit: $100
Estimated new entrants: 176
School starts: Aug. 1987

Approximate Expenses per Year (1985–86):
Tuition: $18,200
Fees: $300
Other costs: $8,900

Statistics (1985–86):
Applicants: 4,250 (2,161 in-state; 2,089 out-of-state)
New entrants: 178 (131 in-state; 47 out-of-state)

Requirements: MCAT, premedical curriculum (bachelor's degree highly recommended).

Required College Courses: Years
Biology (incl. vertebrate zoology; lab)............................1
Inorganic chemistry (with lab) 1
Organic chemistry (with lab) 1
Physics (with lab) 1
English 1

New York University School of Medicine

Office of Admissions
New York University
School of Medicine
P.O. Box 1924
New York, NY 10016   Tel: (212) 430-5290

Application and Acceptance (1987–88):
Application filing: Aug. 15–Dec. 15, 1986
Fee: $50
Notification: Dec. 1, 1986–Aug. 31, 1987
Deposit: $100
Estimated new entrants: 155
School starts: Sept. 1987

Approximate Expenses per Year (1985–86):
Tuition: $13,000
Fees: $1,300
Other costs: $5,000

Statistics (1985–86):
Applicants: 4,038 (3,138 in-state; 900 out-of-state)
New entrants: 156 (122 in-state; 34 out-of-state)
Sex: 33–40% women (average)

Requirements: MCAT, three years of college (bachelor's degree strongly recommended).

Required College Courses: Sem. hrs.
Biology (with lab) 6
Inorganic chemistry (with lab) 6
Organic chemistry (with lab) 6
General physics (with lab)..6
English 6

Recommended College Courses: Genetics, embryology, developmental biology, physical chemistry.

University of Rochester
School of Medicine and Dentistry

Director of Admissions
University of Rochester
School of Medicine and Dentistry
601 Elmwood Avenue, Box 601
Rochester, NY 14642   Tel: (716) 275-4539

Application and Acceptance (1987–88):
Application filing: June 15–Nov. 1, 1986
Fee: $50
Notification from: Oct. 15, 1986
Estimated new entrants: 104
School starts: Sept. 1987

Approximate Expenses per Year (1985–86):
Tuition: $13,300
Fees: $700
Other costs: $6,900

Statistics (1985–86):
Applicants: 2,871 (1,612 in-state; 1,259 out-of-state)
New entrants: 104 (63 in-state; 41 out-of-state)

Requirements: Three years of college (bachelor's degree preferred), preference given to residents of New York State.

Required College Courses:	Years
Biology	1
Chemistry (incl. 1 yr. organic)	2
Physics	1
English	1

State University of New York at Buffalo
School of Medicine

Office of Medical Admissions
Room 138, Farber Hall
State University of New York at Buffalo
School of Medicine
Buffalo, NY 14214   Tel: (716) 831-3466

Application and Acceptance (1987–88):
AMCAS application filing: June 15–Dec. 1, 1986
Fee: $50
Notification: Oct. 1986–Aug. 19, 1987
Deposit: $100
Estimated new entrants: 135
School starts: Aug. 1987

Approximate Expenses per Year (1985–86):
Tuition: $5,600 (resident); $8,300 (nonresident)
Fees: $400
Other costs: $8,500

Statistics (1985–86):
Applicants: 3,132 (2,682 in-state; 450 out-of-state)
New entrants: 135 (132 in-state; 3 out-of-state)

Requirements: MCAT, bachelor's degree recommended, preference given to New York State residents.

Required College Courses: Years
Biology (zoology or botany/zoology; lab)......................................1
General or inorganic chemistry (with lab) 1
Organic chemistry (with lab)..½
General physics 1
English 1

Recommended College Courses: Mathematics (incl. calculus), embryology, genetics, quantitative and physical chemistry.

State University of New York Downstate Medical Center College of Medicine

Office of Admissions, Box 60
State University of New York
Downstate Medical Center
450 Clarkson Avenue
Brooklyn, NY 11203-9967   Tel: (212) 270-2735

Application and Acceptance (1987–88):
AMCAS application filing: June 15–Dec. 1, 1986
Fee: $50
Notification from: Oct. 15, 1986
Estimated new entrants: 200
School starts: Sept. 1987

Approximate Expenses per Year (1985–86):
Tuition: $5,500 (resident); $8,900 (nonresident)
Fees: $100
Other costs: $5,600

Statistics (1985–86):
Applicants: 3,504 (2,867 in-state; 637 out-of-state)
New entrants: 199 (191 in-state; 8 out-of-state)
Mean GPA: 3.51
Sex: 33.7% women; 66.3% men

Requirements: MCAT, three years of college (bachelor's degree recommended), preference given to New York State residents.

Required College Courses: Years
General biology or zoology (with lab) 1
Inorganic chemistry (with lab) 1
Organic chemistry (with lab) 1
General physics (with lab) 1
English 1

Recommended College Courses: Mathematics, advanced-level science.

State University of New York at Stony Brook
Health Sciences Center
School of Medicine

Committee on Admissions
Level 4, Room 046
State University of New York at Stony Brook
Health Sciences Center
School of Medicine
Stony Brook, NY 11794   Tel: (516) 444-2113

Application and Acceptance (1987–88):
Application filing: July 1–Dec. 15, 1986
Fee: $50
Notification from: Oct. 1986
Estimated new entrants: 100
School starts: Sept. 1987

Approximate Expenses per Year (1985–86):
Tuition: $5,600 (resident); $8,400 (nonresident)
Fees: $100
Other costs: $7,000

Statistics (1985–86):
Applicants: 2,397
New entrants: 100 (99 in-state; 1 out-of-state)

Requirements: MCAT, bachelor's degree generally required.

Required College Courses:	Years
Biology (with lab)	1
Inorganic chemistry (with lab)	1
Organic chemistry (with lab)	1
Physics (with lab)	1
English	1

State University of New York
Upstate Medical Center
College of Medicine

Admissions Committee
State University of New York
Upstate Medical Center
College of Medicine
155 Elizabeth Blackwell Street
Syracuse, NY 13210   Tel: (315) 473-4570

Application and Acceptance (1987–88):
AMCAS application filing: June 15–Dec. 15, 1986
Fee: $50
Notification: Oct. 15, 1986–Aug. 30, 1987
Deposit: $100
Estimated new entrants: 150
School starts: Aug. 1987

Approximate Expenses per Year (1985–86):
Tuition: $5,600 (resident); $8,900 (nonresident)
Fees: $100
Other costs: $6,400

Statistics (1985–86):
Applicants: 3,321 (2,827 in-state; 494 out-of-state)
New entrants: 150 (127 in-state; 23 out-of-state)
Mean GPA: 3.56
Sex: 38.6% women; 61.4% men

Requirements: MCAT, three years of college (90 sem. hrs.), preference given to New York State residents.

Required College Courses: Sem. hrs.
Chemistry, inorganic (with lab) 6–8
             organic (with lab) 6–8
Biology or zoology (with lab) 6–8
Physics (with lab) 6–8
English 6

Bowman Gray School of Medicine of Wake Forest University

Office of Medical School Admissions
Bowman Gray School of Medicine
  of Wake Forest University
300 South Hawthorne Road
Winston-Salem, NC 27103   Tel: (919) 748-4264

Application and Acceptance (1987–88):
AMCAS application filing: June 15–Nov. 1, 1986
Fee: $40
Notification: Oct. 15, 1986–April 15, 1987
Deposit: $100
Estimated new entrants: 108
School starts: Aug. 1987

Approximate Expenses per Year (1985–86):
Tuition and fees: $9,000
Other costs: $7,500

Statistics (1985–86):
Applicants: 3,645 (508 in-state; 3,137 out-of-state)
New entrants: 108 (65 in-state; 43 out-of-state)
Sex: 35% women; 65% men

Requirements: MCAT, 90 sem. hrs. of college work (bachelor's
  degree recommended).

Required College Courses:	Sem. hrs.
General biology	8
General or inorganic chemistry	8
Organic chemistry	8
General physics	8

Recommended College Courses: Biochemistry, zoology,
  English, social and behavioral sciences.

Duke University School of Medicine

Committee on Admissions
Duke University
School of Medicine
Duke University Medical Center
P.O. Box 3710
Durham, NC 27710   Tel: (919) 684-2985

Application and Acceptance (1987–88):
Application request until: Oct. 15, 1986
Application filing: June 1–Nov. 1, 1986
Fee: $45
Notification from: Oct. 15, 1986
Deposit: $50
Estimated new entrants: 114
School starts: Aug. 1987

Approximate Expenses per Year (1985–86):
Tuition: $10,500
Fees: $600
Other costs: $7,800

Statistics (1985–86):
Applicants: 3,118 (215 in-state; 2,903 out-of-state)
New entrants: 112 (30 in-state; 82 out-of-state)
Sex: 29% women; 71% men

Requirements: MCAT, three years of college (90 sem. hrs.).

Required College Courses:	Years
Biology and/or zoology	1
Inorganic chemistry	1
Organic chemistry	1
General physics	1
Calculus	1
English	1

Recommended College Courses: Embryology, physical chemistry, biochemistry.

East Carolina University School of Medicine

Associate Dean
Office of Admissions and Student Affairs
East Carolina University
School of Medicine
Greenville, NC 27834   Tel: (919) 757-2202

Application and Acceptance (1987–88):
AMCAS application filing: June 15–Dec. 1, 1986
Fee: $15
Offers Early Decision Plan (residents only)
    EDP application filing: June 15–Aug. 1, 1986
    Notification by: Oct. 1, 1986
Regular applicants notified from: Oct. 15, 1986
Deposit: $100
Estimated new entrants: 64
School starts: Aug. 1987

Approximate Expenses per Year (1985–86):
Tuition: $1,100 (resident); $3,600 (nonresident)
Fees: $300
Other costs: $5,500

Statistics (1985–86):
Applicants: 948 (581 in-state; 367 out-of-state)
New entrants: 64 (63 in-state; 1 out-of-state)
Mean GPA: 3.3
Sex: 33% women; 67% men

Requirements: MCAT, three years of college (bachelor's degree
    recommended), preference given to North Carolina residents.

Required College Courses: Years
General biology or zoology (with lab) 1
Inorganic chemistry (with lab) 1
Organic chemistry (with lab) 1
Physics (with lab) 1
English 1

Recommended College Courses: Humanities, social sciences,
    upper-level English.

University of North Carolina at Chapel Hill
School of Medicine

Committee on Admissions
121 MacNider Hall 202-H
University of North Carolina at Chapel Hill
School of Medicine
Chapel Hill, NC 27514   Tel: (919) 962-8331

Application and Acceptance (1987–88):
AMCAS application filing: June 15–Nov. 15, 1986
Fee: $15
Offers Early Decision Plan
    EDP application filing: June 15–Aug. 1, 1986
    Notification by: Oct. 1, 1986
Regular applicants notified from: Oct. 15, 1986
Deposit: $100
Estimated new entrants: 160
School starts: Aug. 1987

Approximate Expenses per Year (1985–86):
Tuition: $2,100 (resident); $6,200 (nonresident)
Fees: $300
Other costs: $4,700

Statistics (1985–86):
Applicants: 2,091 (617 in-state; 1,474 out-of-state)
New entrants: 160 (140 in-state; 20 out-of-state)

Requirements: MCAT, 96 sem. hrs. of college credit, prefer-
    ence given to North Carolina residents.

Required College Courses: Sem. hrs.
Biology (incl. vertebrate zoology; lab) 8
Chemistry (inorganic and organic, incl. qualitative and
    quantitative analysis; lab) 16
General physics (with lab) 8
English 6

Recommended College Courses: Advanced biology, chemistry,
    and mathematics.

University of North Dakota School of Medicine

Secretary, Committee on Admissions
University of North Dakota
School of Medicine
501 Columbia Road
Grand Forks, ND 58201   Tel: (701) 777-4221

Application and Acceptance (1987–88):
Application filing: July 1–Nov. 1, 1986
Fee: $15
Notification from: Jan. 1, 1987
Deposit: $75
Estimated new entrants: 55
School starts: Aug. 1987

Approximate Expenses per Year (1985–86):
Tuition: $2,600 (resident); $5,200 (nonresident)
Fees: $200
Other costs: $7,400 (resident); $7,400 (nonresident)

Statistics (1985–86):
Applicants: 136 (115 in-state; 21 out-of-state)
New entrants: 55 (51 in-state; 4 out-of-state)
Mean GPA: 3.0 (minimum)

Requirements: MCAT, three years of college (90 sem. hrs.), bachelor's degree recommended, strong preference given to qualified North Dakota residents.

Required College Courses: Sem. hrs.
General biology (incl. zoology) 8
Inorganic and qualitative chemistry 8
Organic chemistry 8
General physics 8
Algebra 3
Psychology/sociology 3
English/communications 6

Recommended College Courses: Computer science.

Case Western Reserve University School of Medicine

Office of Admissions
Case Western Reserve University
School of Medicine
2119 Abington Road
Cleveland, OH 44106   Tel: (216) 368-3450

Application and Acceptance (1987–88):
AMCAS application filing: June 15–Nov. 1, 1986
Fee: $30
Offers Early Decision Plan (residents only)
 EDP application filing: June 15–Aug. 1, 1986
 Notification by: Oct. 1, 1986
Regular applicants notified: Oct. 15, 1986–May 15, 1987
Estimated new entrants: 138
School starts: Aug. 1987

Approximate Expenses per Year (1985–86):
Tuition: $12,300
Fees: $700
Other costs: $12,100

Statistics (1985–86):
Applicants: 5,583 (1,030 in-state; 4,553 out-of-state)
New entrants: 138 (83 in-state; 55 out-of-state)

Requirements: MCAT, three years of college.

Required College Courses:	Years
Biology	1
General or inorganic chemistry	1
Organic chemistry	1
Physics	1
English	1

Recommended College Courses: Mathematics (incl. calculus).

University of Cincinnati College of Medicine

Office of Student Affairs
Mail Location #552
University of Cincinnati
College of Medicine
231 Bethesda Avenue
Cincinnati, OH 45267   Tel: (513) 872-7314

Application and Acceptance (1987–88):
AMCAS application filing: June 15–Nov. 15, 1986
Fee: $25
Offers Early Decision Plan
    EDP application filing: June 15–Aug. 1, 1986
    Notification by: Oct. 1, 1986
Regular applicants notified: Oct. 15, 1986–Sept. 10, 1987
Estimated new entrants: 192
School starts: Sept. 1987

Approximate Expenses per Year (1985–86):
Tuition: $5,300 (resident); $8,300 (nonresident)
Fees: $400
Other costs: $7,600

Statistics (1985–86):
Applicants: 4,059 (1,315 in-state; 2,744 out-of-state)
New entrants: 192 (152 in-state; 40 out-of-state)
Mean GPA: 3.5
Sex: 31% women; 69% men

Requirements: MCAT, three years of college (bachelor's degree recommended), preference given to Ohio residents.

Required College Courses: Years
General biology (with lab)..1
General or inorganic chemistry (with lab) 1
Organic chemistry (with lab) 1
General physics (with lab)..1
English 1

Recommended College Courses: Advanced biology, mathematics, English, history, psychology, sociology, logic, philosophy.

Medical College of Ohio at Toledo

Admissions Office
Medical College of Ohio at Toledo
Caller Service No. 10008
Toledo, OH 43699   Tel: (419) 381-4229

Application and Acceptance (1987–88):
AMCAS application filing: June 15–Nov. 1, 1986
Fee: $30
Offers Early Decision Plan (residents only)
    EDP application filing: June 15–Aug. 1, 1986
    Notification by: Oct. 1, 1986
Regular applicants notified from: Oct. 15, 1986
Estimated new entrants: 150
School starts: Aug. 1987

Approximate Expenses per Year (1985–86):
Tuition: $5,400 (resident); $6,900 (nonresident)
Fees: $200
Other costs: $9,500

Statistics (1985–86):
Applicants: 1,200 (860 in-state; 340 out-of-state)
New entrants: 150 (145 in-state; 5 out-of-state)
Mean GPA: 3.43
Sex: 30% women; 70% men

Requirements: MCAT, bachelor's degree recommended, preference given to Ohio residents.

Required College Courses: Years
Biology 1
Inorganic chemistry 1
Organic chemistry 1
Physics 1
Mathematics 1

Recommended College Courses: Advanced biology, English.

Northeastern Ohio Universities College of Medicine

Admissions Program
Office of Student Affairs
Northeastern Ohio Universities
College of Medicine
Rootstown, OH 44272 Tel: (216) 325-2511

Application and Acceptance (1987–88):
AMCAS application filing: June 15–Nov. 1, 1986
Fee: $20
Offers Early Decision Plan
    EDP application filing: June 15–Aug. 1, 1986
    Notification by: Oct. 1, 1986
Regular applicants notified from: Oct. 15, 1986
Estimated new entrants: 10 (4-yr. M.D. degree program; does
    not include combined B.S./M.D. program students)
School starts: Sept. 1987

Approximate Expenses per Year (1985–86):
Tuition: $3,800 (resident); $7,500 (nonresident)
Fees: $700
Other costs: $5,100

Statistics (1985–86):
Applicants: 869 (744 in-state; 125 out-of-state)
New entrants: 22 (21 in-state; 1 out-of-state)

Requirements: MCAT, three years of college, preference given
    to Ohio residents. (B.S./M.D. program admission restricted
    to students who have taken no college course work follow-
    ing high school graduation.)

Required College Courses: Years
Organic chemistry 1
Physics 1

Recommended College Courses: General chemistry, general
    biology, embryology, physiology, microbiology, sociology,
    psychology, biochemistry, statistics, calculus, humanities.

Ohio State University College of Medicine

Admissions Committee
Room 270-A, Meling Hall
Ohio State University
College of Medicine
370 West Ninth Avenue
Columbus, OH 43210   Tel: (614) 422-7137

Application and Acceptance (1987–88):
AMCAS application filing: June 15–Nov. 15, 1986
Fee: $10
Offers Early Decision Plan
       EDP application filing: June 15–Aug. 1, 1986
       Notification by: Oct. 1, 1986
Regular applicants notified from: Oct. 15, 1986
Estimated new entrants: 233
School starts: Sept. 1987

Approximate Expenses per Year (1985–86):
Tuition (3 qtrs.): $3,900 (resident); $8,400 (nonresident)
Fees: $120
Other costs: $4,900

Statistics (1985–86):
Applicants: 2,060 (1,200 in-state; 860 out-of-state)
New entrants: 233 (210 in-state; 23 out-of-state)
Mean GPA: 3.5

Requirements: MCAT, bachelor's degree, preference given to
       Ohio residents.

Required College Courses: Years
Biology (incl. vertebrate zoology) 1
Inorganic chemistry (with lab) 1
Organic chemistry (with lab)..1
General physics (with lab) 1

Recommended College Courses: History, art, literature, cre-
       ative writing, philosophy, social sciences, communications.

Wright State University School of Medicine

Office of Student Affairs/Admissions
Wright State University
School of Medicine
P.O. Box 1751
Dayton, OH 45401   Tel: (513) 873-2934

Application and Acceptance (1987–88):
AMCAS application filing: June 15–Nov. 15, 1986
Fee: $25
Offers Early Decision Plan
    EDP application filing: June 15–Aug. 1, 1986
    Notification by: Oct. 1, 1986
Regular applicants notified from: Oct. 15, 1986
Estimated new entrants: 100
School starts: Sept. 1987

Approximate Expenses per Year (1985–86):
Tuition: $5,400 (resident); $8,000 (nonresident)
Fees: $300
Other costs: $7,300

Statistics (1985–86):
Applicants: 1,573 (1,078 in-state; 495 out-of-state)
New entrants: 100 (98 in-state; 2 out-of-state)

Requirements: MCAT, three years of college (90 sem./135 qtr. hrs.), preference given to Ohio residents.

Required College Courses: Years
Biology 1
Chemistry (incl. organic)...2
Physics 1
Mathematics 1
English 1

University of Oklahoma College of Medicine

Director of Admissions
Room 357, Biomedical Sciences Building
University of Oklahoma
College of Medicine
P.O. Box 26901
Oklahoma City, OK 73190   Tel: (405) 271-2339

Application and Acceptance (1987–88):
AMCAS application filing: June 15–Nov. 1, 1986
Fee: $10 (residents); $15 (nonresidents)
Notification from: Oct. 15, 1986
Deposit: $100
Estimated new entrants: 176
School starts: Aug. 1987

Approximate Expenses per Year (1985–86):
Tuition: $2,100 (resident); $5,100 (nonresident)
Fees: $200
Other costs: $6,900

Statistics (1985–86):
Applicants: 850 (312 in-state; 538 out-of-state)
New entrants: 176 (164 in-state; 12 out-of-state)
Mean GPA: 3.61
Sex: 21% women; 79% men

Requirements: MCAT, 90 sem. hrs. of college credit (bachelor's degree highly recommended), preference given to residents of Oklahoma.

Required College Courses: Semesters
Vertebrate zoology (with lab) 1
Embryology, genetics, comparative anatomy, cellular
    biology, histology 1
Inorganic (general) chemistry 2
Organic chemistry 2
General physics..2
English..3
Psychology, sociology, anthropology, humanities, political
    science, foreign language, and/or philosophy.....................3

Recommended College Courses: American or English literature.

Oral Roberts University School of Medicine

Office of Graduate Admissions
Oral Roberts University
School of Medicine
7777 South Lewis Avenue
Tulsa, OK 74171   Tel: (918) 495-6514

Application and Acceptance (1987–88):
AMCAS application filing: June 15–Nov. 1, 1986
Fee: $30
Offers Early Decision Plan
    EDP application filing: June 15–Aug. 1, 1986
    Notification by: Oct. 1, 1986
Regular applicants notified from: Oct. 15, 1986
Deposit: $100
Estimated new entrants: 48
School starts: Aug. 1987

Approximate Expenses per Year (1985–86):
Tuition: $8,500
Fees: $300
Other costs: $6,800

Statistics (1985–86):
Applicants: 1,387
New entrants: 48 (0 in-state; 48 out-of-state)
Average GPA: 3.6
Sex: 12.5% women; 87.5% men

Requirements: MCAT, 90 sem. hrs. (135 qtr. hrs.) of college
    credit, bachelor's degree highly desirable.

Required College Courses:	Sem./Qtr.
General biology (with lab)	2/3
General or inorganic chemistry (with lab)	2/3
Organic chemistry (with lab)	2/3
Physics (with lab)	2/3
English	2/3
Calculus I	1/1
General psychology	1/1

Recommended College Courses: Genetics, statistics, compara-
    tive anatomy or vertebrate biology with dissection, physical
    chemistry, advanced-level psychology (2 sem.).

Oregon Health Sciences University School of Medicine

Director of Admissions, L-109A
Oregon Health Sciences University
School of Medicine
3181 S.W. Sam Jackson Park Road
Portland, OR 97201   Tel: (503) 225-7800

Application and Acceptance (1987–88):
AMCAS application filing: June 15–Nov. 15, 1986
Fee: $25
Notification from: March 1, 1987
Estimated new entrants: 90
School starts: Sept. 1987

Approximate Expenses per Year (1985–86):
Tuition: $4,100 (resident); $8,800 (nonresident)
Fees: $500
Other costs: $6,000

Statistics (1985–86):
Applicants: 676 (339 in-state; 337 out-of-state)
New entrants: 90 (90 in-state; 0 out-of-state)
Mean GPA: 3.56

Requirements: MCAT, three years of college (138 qtr./92 sem. hrs.), bachelor's degree recommended, preference given to residents of Oregon and Western states having no medical schools.

Required College Courses: Qtr. hrs.
General biology or zoology (incl. basic genetics) 9
Chemistry 24
    general or inorganic (with lab) 10–16
    organic (with lab) 8–12
General physics (incl. mechanics, heat and sound, light
    and electricity; lab) 12
Mathematics (incl. calculus) 12
General psychology 6

Recommended College Courses: Advanced physiology, embryology, analytical chemistry, instructional analysis, physical chemistry, major modern foreign language.

Hahnemann University School of Medicine

Admissions Office
Mail Stop 442
Hahnemann University
School of Medicine
245 North 15th Street
Philadelphia, PA 19102   Tel: (215) 448-7600

Application and Acceptance (1987–88):
AMCAS application filing: June 15–Nov. 15, 1986
Fee: $50
Offers Early Decision Plan
    EDP application filing: June 15–Aug. 1, 1986
    Notification by: Oct. 1, 1986
Regular applicants notified from: Oct. 15, 1986
Deposit: $100
Estimated new entrants: 165   School starts: Aug. 1987

Approximate Expenses per Year (1985–86):
Tuition: $14,700
Fees: $500
Other costs: $6,800

Statistics (1985–86):
Applicants: 5,820 (1,222 in-state; 4,598 out-of-state)
New entrants: 165 (99 in-state; 66 out-of-state)
Average GPA: 3.4   Sex: 30% women; 70% men

Requirements: MCAT, three years of college (90 sem. hrs.),
    bachelor's degree strongly recommended, preference given
    to Pennsylvania residents.

Required College Courses: Sem. hrs.
General biology (with lab) 8
General or inorganic chemistry (with lab) 8
Organic chemistry (with lab) 8
General physics (with lab) 8
English (composition and literature) 6
Social science 6
Humanities 6

Recommended College Courses: Mathematics, embryology, mam-
    malian comparative anatomy, physical chemistry, quantita-
    tive analysis.

Jefferson Medical College
of Thomas Jefferson University

Associate Dean for Admissions
Jefferson Medical College
    of Thomas Jefferson University
1025 Walnut Street
Philadelphia, PA 19107   Tel: (215) 928-6983

Application and Acceptance (1987–88):
AMCAS application filing: June 15–Nov. 15, 1986
Fee: $60
Offers Early Decision Plan
    EDP application filing: June 15–Aug. 1, 1986
    Notification by: Oct. 1, 1986
Regular applicants notified from: Oct. 15, 1986
Deposit: $100
Estimated new entrants: 223
School starts: Sept. 1987

Approximate Expenses per Year (1985–86):
Tuition: $13,200
Fees: $100
Other costs: $8,200

Statistics (1985–86):
Applicants: 4,567 (1,438 in-state; 3,129 out-of-state)
New entrants: 223 (125 in-state; 98 out-of-state)
Mean GPA: science, 3.5; nonscience, 3.56
Sex: 26% women; 74% men

Requirements: MCAT, three years of college (90 sem. hrs.),
    bachelor's degree strongly recommended, preference given
    to Pennsylvania residents.

Required College Courses: Years
General biology (with lab)..1
Inorganic chemistry (with lab) 1
Organic chemistry (with lab) 1
General physics (with lab)...1

Medical College of Pennsylvania

Associate Dean for Admissions
Medical College of Pennsylvania
3300 Henry Avenue
Philadelphia, PA 19129   Tel: (215) 842-7009

Application and Acceptance (1987–88):
AMCAS application filing: June 15–Dec. 1, 1986
Fee: $50
Offers Early Decision Plan
    EDP application filing: June 15–Aug. 1, 1986
    Notification by: Oct. 1, 1986
Regular applicants notified from: Oct. 15, 1986
Deposit: $100
Estimated new entrants: 100
School starts: Sept. 1987

Approximate Expenses per Year (1985–86):
Tuition: $12,500
Fees: $900
Other costs: $8,200

Statistics (1985–86):
Applicants: 4,243 (1,404 in-state; 2,839 out-of-state)
New entrants: 100 (74 in-state; 26 out-of-state)
Average GPA: 3.48

Requirements: MCAT, 90 sem. hrs. of college credit (bachelor's
    degree highly recommended).

Required College Courses: Sem.
Biology (with lab) 2
Inorganic chemistry (with lab) 2
Organic chemistry (with lab) 2
General physics (with lab)..2
English 2

Pennsylvania State University College of Medicine

Office of Student Affairs
Pennsylvania State University
College of Medicine
P.O. Box 850
Hershey, PA 17033   Tel: (717) 534-8755

Application and Acceptance (1987–88):
AMCAS application filing: June–Nov. 15, 1986
Fee: $40
Notification from: Oct. 15, 1986
Deposit: $100
Estimated new entrants: 95
School starts: Sept. 1987

Approximate Expenses per Year (1985–86):
Tuition: $8,100 (resident); $12,700 (nonresident)
Fees: $300
Other costs: $8,400

Statistics (1985–86):
Applicants: 1,427 (929 in-state; 498 out-of-state)
New entrants: 95 (80 in-state; 15 out-of-state)
Average GPA: 3.6
Sex: 30% women; 70% men

Requirements: MCAT, three years of college (bachelor's degree highly desirable), preference given to Pennsylvania residents.

Required College Courses: Years
Biology 1
Inorganic chemistry 1
Organic chemistry 1
Physics 1

Recommended College Courses: Mathematics (calculus), behavioral science, genetics, physical chemistry.

University of Pennsylvania School of Medicine

Director of Admissions
Suite 100, 1st Floor, Medical Education Building
University of Pennsylvania
School of Medicine (GM)
Philadelphia, PA 19104   Tel: (215) 898-8001

Application and Acceptance (1987–88):
AMCAS application filing: June 15–Nov. 1, 1986
Fee: $50
Notification from: Dec. 1, 1986
Deposit: $100
Estimated new entrants: 155
School starts: Aug. 1987

Approximate Expenses per Year (1985–86):
Tuition: $13,100
Fees: $600
Other costs: $8,800

Statistics (1985–86):
Applicants: 5,739 (1,118 in-state; 4,621 out-of-state)
New entrants: 156 (70 in-state; 86 out-of-state)

Requirements: MCAT, bachelor's degree.

Required College Courses: Years
General biology (with lab)..1
Inorganic chemistry (with lab) 1
Organic chemistry (with lab) 1
Physics (with lab) 1

University of Pittsburgh School of Medicine

Office of Admissions
M-245 Scaife Hall
University of Pittsburgh
School of Medicine
Pittsburgh, PA 15261   Tel: (412) 624-2489

Application and Acceptance (1987–88):
AMCAS application filing: June 15–Nov. 1, 1986
Fee: $40
Offers Early Decision Plan
    EDP application filing: June 15–Aug. 1, 1986
    Notification by: Oct. 1, 1986
Regular applicants notified from: Nov. 15, 1986
Estimated new entrants: 136
School starts: Sept. 1987

Approximate Expenses per Year (1985–86):
Tuition: $12,100 (resident); $16,900 (nonresident)
Fees: $100
Other costs: $12,000

Statistics (1985–86):
Applicants: 3,062 (1,143 in-state; 1,919 out-of-state)
New entrants: 136 (94 in-state; 42 out-of-state)

Requirements: MCAT, bachelor's degree strongly recommended, some preference given to Pennsylvania residents.

Required College Courses: Years
Biology (excl. of botany; lab) 1
Inorganic chemistry (with lab) 1
Organic chemistry (with lab) 1
Physics (with lab) 1
Calculus 1
English (composition and literature) 1
Psychology, sociology, and/or anthropology 1

Temple University School of Medicine

Admissions Office
Suite 305, Student Faculty Center
Temple University
School of Medicine
Broad and Ontario Streets
Philadelphia, PA 19140   Tel: (215) 221-3656

Application and Acceptance (1987–88):
AMCAS application filing: June 15–Dec. 1, 1986
Fee: $35
Offers Early Decision Plan
    EDP application filing: June 15–Aug. 1, 1986
    Notification by: Sept. 1, 1986
Regular applicants notified from: Oct. 15, 1986–Aug. 15, 1987
Deposit: $100
Estimated new entrants: 180
School starts: Sept. 1987

Approximate Expenses per Year (1985–86):
Tuition: $9,300 (resident); $12,600 (nonresident)
Fees: $200
Other costs: $7,200

Statistics (1985–86):
Applicants: 4,178 (1,446 in-state; 2,732 out-of-state)
New entrants: 172 (140 in-state; 32 out-of-state)
Mean GPA: 3.4
Sex: 35% women; 65% men

Requirements: MCAT, 90 sem. hrs. of college credit, prefer-
    ence given to residents of Pennsylvania.

Required College Courses: Years
Biology (with lab) 1
Inorganic chemistry (with lab) 1
Organic chemistry (with lab) 1
General physics (with lab) 1

Universidad Central del Caribe School of Medicine

Section on Admissions
Office of the Dean
Universidad Central del Caribe
School of Medicine
156 Munoz Rivera
Cayey, PR 00633   Tel: (809) 738-3013

Application and Acceptance (1986–87):
Application filing: Jan 1, 1986 (*July 1, 1986**)–April 15, 1986
   (*Oct. 15, 1986**)
Fee: $50
Notification: June 1, 1986 (*Dec. 1, 1986**)–Aug. 1, 1986 (*Jan. 15, 1987**)
Estimated new entrants: 80
School starts: Aug. 1986 (*Jan. 1987**)

Approximate Expenses per Year (1984–85):
Tuition: $13,000 (resident); $15,000 (nonresident)
Fees: $100
Other costs: $2,400

Statistics (1984–85):
Applicants: 335 (223 Puerto Rico; 112 other)
New entrants: 80 (61 Puerto Rico; 19 other)
Mean GPA: 3.04
Sex: 29% women; 71% men

Requirements: MCAT, 90 college credits, proficiency in both
   Spanish and English.

Required College Courses:	Sem. hrs.
General biology or zoology	8
General chemistry	8
Organic chemistry	8
General physics	8
Mathematics	6
English	6
Spanish	6

Recommended College Courses: Social sciences, humanities.

*Dates in italics refer to class entering January 1987.

Ponce School of Medicine

Admissions Office
Ponce School of Medicine
P.O. Box 7004
Ponce, PR 00732   Tel: (809) 840-2575

Application and Acceptance (1987–88):
AMCAS application filing: June 15–Dec. 15, 1986
Fee: $25
Notification from: Dec. 1, 1986
Deposit: $1,000
Estimated new entrants: 50
School starts: July 1987

Approximate Expenses per Year (1985–86):
Tuition: $11,000 (resident); $13,000 (nonresident)
Fees: $300
Other costs: $10,400 (resident); $11,100 (nonresident)

Statistics (1985–86):
Applicants: 734 (193 Puerto Rico; 541 other)
New entrants: 40 (30 Puerto Rico; 10 other)
Average GPA: 3.27
Sex: 23% women; 77% men

Requirements: MCAT, three years of college (90 sem. hrs.),
  preference given to residents of Puerto Rico.

Required College Courses: Sem. hrs.
Biology 8
Inorganic chemistry 8
Organic chemistry 8
Physics 8
Algebra 3
Trigonometry 3
Humanities 6
English 12
Spanish 12

University of Puerto Rico School of Medicine

Central Admissions Office
University of Puerto Rico
School of Medicine
Medical Sciences Campus
G.P.O. Box 5067
San Juan, PR 00936   Tel: (809) 753-2966

Application and Acceptance (1987–88):
Application filing: July 1–Dec. 15, 1986
Fee: $15
Notification: March 1–May 15, 1987
Deposit: $25
Estimated new entrants: 150
School starts: Aug. 1987

Approximate Expenses per Year (1985–86):
Tuition: $2,300 (resident); standardized fee scale for nonresidents
Fees: $200
Other costs: $5,500

Statistics (1985–86):
Applicants: 506 (465 Puerto Rico; 41 other)
New entrants: 151 (149 Puerto Rico; 2 other)
Mean GPA: 3.45
Sex: 36% women; 64% men

Requirements: MCAT, 90 sem. hrs. of college credit, fluency in
   Spanish and English, preference given to residents of
   Puerto Rico.

Required College Courses:	Credits
Biology (with lab)	8
Inorganic chemistry (with lab)	8
Organic chemistry (with lab)	8
Physics (with lab)	8
English	12
Spanish	12
Behavioral and social sciences (sociology, psychology, political sciences, economics, anthropology)	6

Recommended College Courses: Mathematics.

Brown University Program in Medicine

Office of Admission
Box G
Brown University
Program in Medicine
Providence, RI 02912   Tel: (401) 863-2149

Application and Acceptance (1987–88):
Application filing: Aug. 15–Nov. 1, 1986
Fee: $60
Offers Early Decision Plan
    EDP application filing: July 1–Aug. 15, 1986
    Notification by: Oct. 1, 1986
Regular applicants notified from: Nov. 1, 1986
Deposit: $100
Estimated new entrants: 60 (majority from the 7-yr. continuum
    program)
School starts: Sept. 1987

Approximate Expenses per Year (1985–86):
Tuition: $12,300
Fees: $400
Other costs: $6,000

Statistics (1985–86):
Applicants: 1,103 (87 in-state; 1,016 out-of-state)
New entrants: 61 (19 in-state; 42 out-of-state)

Requirements: MCAT, three years of college (bachelor's degree
    preferred).

> NOTE: There will be no regular admissions to Brown's
> medical program for 1987–88. All students will be
> coming through the 7- to 8-year continuum.

Required College Courses: Sem.
Biology 3
Biochemistry 1
General chemistry 2
Organic chemistry 2
Physics 2
Calculus 2
Behavioral or social sciences 3

Recommended College Courses: Molecular biology, cell physi-
    ology, histology.

Medical University of South Carolina College of Medicine

University Registrar and
Director of Admissions
Medical University of South Carolina
College of Medicine
171 Ashley Avenue
Charleston, SC 29425   Tel: (803) 792-3281

Application and Acceptance (1987–88):
AMCAS application filing: June 15–Dec. 1, 1986
Fee: $15
Offers Early Decision Plan (residents only)
    EDP application filing: June 15–Aug. 1, 1986
    Notification by: Oct. 1, 1986
Regular applicants notified from: Oct. 15, 1986
Deposit: $50
Estimated new entrants: 155
School starts: Aug. 1987

Approximate Expenses per Year (1985–86):
Tuition and fees: $3,300 (resident); $6,600 (nonresident)
Other costs: $10,600 (resident); $13,900 (nonresident)

Statistics (1985–86):
Applicants: 1,004 (376 in-state; 628 out-of-state)
New entrants: 165 (159 in-state; 6 out-of-state)

Requirements: MCAT, three years of college (90 sem. hrs.),
    bachelor's degree preferred.

Required College Courses: No specific course requirements.

University of South Carolina School of Medicine

Director, Office of Admissions
University of South Carolina
School of Medicine
Columbia, SC 29208   Tel: (803) 733-3325

Application and Acceptance (1987–88):
AMCAS application filing: June 15–Dec. 1, 1986
Fee: $20
Offers Early Decision Plan
    EDP application filing: June 15–Aug. 1, 1986
    Notification by: Oct. 1, 1986
Regular applicants notified from: Oct. 15, 1986
Deposit: $100
Estimated new entrants: 64
School starts: Aug. 1987

Approximate Expenses per Year (1985–86):
Tuition and fees: $3,000 (resident); $6,000 (nonresident)
Other costs: $7,900

Statistics (1985–86):
Applicants: 619 (328 in-state; 291 out-of-state)
New entrants: 64 (54 in-state; 10 out-of-state)

Requirements: MCAT, three years of college (bachelor's degree recommended), preference given to residents of South Carolina.

Required College Courses: Years
General biology or zoology (with lab) 1
Inorganic chemistry (with lab) 1
Organic chemistry (with lab) 1
General physics (with lab)..1
Algebra...1
English (composition and literature) 1

Recommended College Courses: Integral and differential calculus.

University of South Dakota School of Medicine

Office of Student Affairs
University of South Dakota
School of Medicine
Vermillion, SD 57069   Tel: (605) 677-5233

Application and Acceptance (1987–88):
AMCAS application filing: June 15–Nov. 15, 1986
Fee: $15 (after screening)
Notification: Dec. 15, 1986–March 15, 1987
Deposit: $250
Estimated new entrants: 50
School starts: Aug. 1987

Approximate Expenses per Year (1985–86):
Tuition: $5,500 (resident); $11,400 (nonresident)
Fees: $600
Other costs: $10,000

Statistics (1985–86):
Applicants: 313 (95 in-state; 218 out-of-state)
New entrants: 50 (48 in-state; 2 out-of-state)
Mean GPA: 3.62
Sex: 30% women; 70% men

Requirements: MCAT, three years of college (90 sem. hrs.), bachelor's degree recommended, preference given to residents of South Dakota.

Required College Courses: Sem. hrs.
General biology or zoology (with lab) 8
General chemistry (incl. qualitative analysis; lab) 8–10
Organic chemistry (incl. aliphatic and aromatic
    compounds; lab) 6–8
Quantitative analysis 2
General physics (with lab) 8
Mathematics (analytical geometry and calculus) 8
English (composition and literature) 12
Psychology and sociology 6

Recommended College Courses: Genetics, embryology, computer science.

East Tennessee State University
Quillen–Dishner College of Medicine

Admissions Officer/Registrar
East Tennessee State University
Quillen–Dishner College of Medicine
P.O. Box 19,900A
Johnson City, TN 37614-0002   Tel: (615) 928-6426, Ext. 220

Application and Acceptance (1987–88):
AMCAS application filing: June 15–Dec. 1, 1986
Fee: $15
Offers Early Decision Plan
 EDP application filing: June 15–Aug. 1, 1986
 Notification by: Oct. 1, 1986
Regular applicants notified from: Oct. 15, 1986
Deposit: $100
Estimated new entrants: 54
School starts: Aug. 1987

Approximate Expenses per Year (1985–86):
Tuition: $5,000 (resident); $7,600 (nonresident)
Fees: $200
Other costs: $7,700

Statistics (1985–86):
Applicants: 886 (434 in-state; 452 out-of-state)
New entrants: 56 (55 in-state; 1 out-of-state)
Mean GPA: 3.4
Sex: 35% women; 65% men

Requirements: MCAT, three years of college (90 sem. hrs.), bachelor's degree recommended, preference given to Tennessee residents.

Required College Courses:	Sem. hrs.
Biology (with lab)	8
General or inorganic chemistry (with lab)	8
Organic chemistry (with lab)	8
Physics (with lab)	8
Communications skills	9

Meharry Medical College School of Medicine

Director of Admissions and Records
Meharry Medical College
School of Medicine
1005 D. B. Todd, Jr. Boulevard
Nashville, TN 37208   Tel: (615) 327-6223

Application and Acceptance (1987–88):
AMCAS application filing: June 15–Dec. 15, 1986
Fee: $25
Offers Early Decision Plan
    EDP application filing: June 15–Aug. 1, 1986
    Notification by: Oct. 1, 1986
Regular applicants notified from: Oct. 15, 1986
Deposit: $100
Estimated new entrants: 80
School starts: June and Aug. 1987

Approximate Expenses per Year (1985–86):
Tuition: $8,500
Fees: $800
Other costs: $13,200

Statistics (1985–86):
Applicants: 3,262 (175 in-state; 3,087 out-of-state)
New entrants: 80 (11 in-state; 69 out-of-state)
Sex: 47% women; 53% men

Requirements: MCAT, three years of college (bachelor's degree
    recommended).

Required College Courses:	Sem. hrs./Qtr. hrs.
General biology or zoology (with lab)	8/12
General chemistry (with lab)	8/12
Organic chemistry (with lab)	8/12
General physics (with lab)	8/12
English	6/9

University of Tennessee
Center for the Health Sciences
College of Medicine

Director of Admissions
University of Tennessee
College of Medicine
800 Madison Avenue
Memphis, TN 38163   Tel: (901) 528-5559

Application and Acceptance (1987–88):
Application filing until: Oct. 15, 1986
Fee: $25
Notification: Nov. 1, 1986–April 15, 1987
Deposit: $100
Estimated new entrants: 180
School starts: Sept. 1987

Approximate Expenses per Year (1985–86):
Tuition: $4,800 (resident); $7,500 (nonresident)
Fees: $300
Other costs: $6,000

Statistics (1985–86):
Applicants: 652 (503 in-state; 149 out-of-state)
New entrants: 177 (163 in-state; 14 out-of-state)
Mean GPA: 3.5

Requirements: MCAT, three years of college (90 sem./135 qtr. hrs.), bachelor's degree recommended, preference given to Tennessee residents.

Required College Courses: Qtr. hrs.
Biology (incl. 4 sem./6 qtr. hrs. of zoology; lab) 12
Inorganic chemistry (with lab) 12
Organic chemistry (with lab) 12
General physics (with lab) 12
English (composition and literature) 9
Electives 78

Vanderbilt University School of Medicine

Assistant Dean of Student Services
Vanderbilt University
School of Medicine
Nashville, TN 37232   Tel: (615) 322-2145

Application and Acceptance (1987–88):
AMCAS application filing: June 15–Nov. 1, 1986
Fee: $25
Offers Early Decision Plan
    EDP application filing: June 15–Aug. 1, 1986
    Notification by: Oct. 1, 1986
Regular applicants notified from: Oct. 15, 1986
Deposit: $50
Estimated new entrants: 100
School starts: Aug. 1987

Approximate Expenses per Year (1985–86):
Tuition: $8,900
Fees: $300
Other costs: $6,000

Statistics (1985–86):
Applicants: 5,093 (236 in-state; 4,857 out-of-state)
New entrants: 101 (15 in-state; 86 out-of-state)
Mean GPA: high B level

Requirements: MCAT, bachelor's degree recommended.

Required College Courses:	Sem. hrs.
Biology (general biology, zoology, and biology, max. 4 hrs. botany; 4 hrs. lab)	8
Inorganic chemistry (with 2 hrs. lab)	8
Organic chemistry (incl. aliphatic and aromatic compounds; 2 hrs. lab)	8
Physics (with 2 hrs. lab)	8
English (composition and literature)	6

Baylor College of Medicine

Director of Admissions
Baylor College of Medicine
One Baylor Plaza
Houston, TX 77030   Tel: (713) 799-4841

Application and Acceptance (1987–88):
Application filing: June 15–Nov. 1, 1986
Fee: $35
Offers Early Decision Plan
    EDP application filing: June 15–Aug. 1, 1986
    Notification by: Oct. 1, 1986
Regular applicants notified from: Nov. 15, 1986–Aug. 6, 1987
Deposit: $300
Estimated new entrants: 168
School starts: Aug. 1987

Approximate Expenses per Year (1985–86):
Tuition: $1,200 (resident); $9,000 (nonresident)
Fees: $600
Other costs: $10,000

Statistics (1985–86):
Applicants: 3,007 (1,175 in-state; 1,832 out-of-state)
New entrants: 168 (118 in-state; 50 out-of-state)
Mean GPA: 3.7
Sex: 35% women; 65% men

Requirements: MCAT, 90 sem. hrs. of college credit (bachelor's
    degree recommended).

Required College Courses:	Years
General biology (with lab)	1
Advanced biology (comparative vertebrate anatomy, physiology, genetics, histology)	½
Inorganic chemistry (with lab)	1
Organic chemistry (with lab)	1
General physics (with lab)	1
English	1

Recommended College Courses: Behavioral science.

Texas A&M University College of Medicine

Associate Dean for Student Affairs
Texas A&M University
College of Medicine
College Station, TX 77843   Tel: (409) 845-7743

Application and Acceptance (1987–88):
Application filing: June 1–Nov. 1, 1986
Notification from: Nov. 15, 1986
Estimated new entrants: 48
School starts: Aug. 1987

Approximate Expenses per Year (1985–86):
Tuition: $2,400 (resident); $9,600 (nonresident)
Fees: $700
Other costs: $6,500

Statistics (1985–86):
Applicants: 1,005 (890 in-state; 115 out-of-state)
New entrants: 48 (44 in-state; 4 out-of-state)
Mean GPA: 3.42
Sex: 37% women; 63% men

Requirements: MCAT, 60 sem. hrs. of college credit, preference given to Texas residents.

Required College Courses:	Sem. hrs.
General biology (with lab)	8
Additional biology	4
Inorganic chemistry (with lab)	8
Organic chemistry (with lab)	8
General physics (with lab)	8
Calculus	3
English	6

Texas Tech University Health Sciences Center School of Medicine

Office of Admissions
Texas Tech University
Health Sciences Center
School of Medicine
Lubbock, TX 79430 Tel: (806) 743-2298

Application and Acceptance (1987–88):
Application filing: April 15–Nov. 1, 1986
Fee: $30
Offers Early Decision Plan (residents only)
    EDP application filing: April 15–Aug. 1, 1986
    Notification by: Oct. 1, 1986
Regular applicants notified from: Oct. 15, 1986
Deposit: $100
Estimated new entrants: 100
School starts: Aug. 1987

Approximate Expenses per Year (1985–86):
Tuition: $1,300 (resident); $3,900 (nonresident)
Fees: $500
Other costs: $11,800

Statistics (1985–86):
Applicants: 938 (938 in-state; 0 out-of-state)
New entrants: 100 (100 in-state; 0 out-of-state)
Mean GPA: 3.36
Sex: 28% women; 72% men

Requirements: MCAT, three years of college (90 sem. hrs.), bachelor's degree recommended.

Required College Courses: Years
Biology or zoology (with lab) 2
Inorganic chemistry (with lab) 1
Organic chemistry (with lab) 1
Physics (with lab) 1

Recommended College Courses: Calculus, social sciences, humanities, Spanish.

University of Texas
Southwestern Medical School at Dallas

Office of the Registrar
University of Texas
Health Science Center at Dallas
5323 Harry Hines Boulevard
Dallas, TX 75235   Tel: (214) 688-3606

Application and Acceptance (1987–88):
Application made through the
    University of Texas System, Medical and Dental Applica-
    tion Center, Suite 102, 210 West 6th Street, Austin TX
    78701
Application filing: April 15–Oct. 15, 1986
Application Center fees
    Resident: $35 (plus $5 for each additional school ap-
                  plied to in the University of Texas system)
    Nonresident: $70 (plus $10 for each additional school ap-
                  plied to in the University of Texas system)
Notification: Jan. 15–Aug. 30, 1987
Estimated new entrants: 205
School starts: Aug. 1987

Approximate Expenses per Year (1985–86):
Tuition: $1,300 (resident); $3,900 (nonresident)
Fees: $200
Other costs: $7,100

Statistics (1985–86):
Applicants: 2,561 (1,748 in-state; 813 out-of-state)
New entrants: 205 (185 in-state; 20 out-of-state)

Requirements: MCAT, three years of college (90 sem. hrs.),
    bachelor's degree preferred, preference given to Texas
    residents.

Required College Courses: Years
Biology (1 yr. lab)..2
Inorganic chemistry (with lab) 1
Organic chemistry (with lab) 1
Physics (with lab) 1
Calculus ....½
English...1

University of Texas Medical School at Galveston

Office of the Registrar and Admissions
Suite 120
Thompson Basic Science Building
University of Texas Medical Branch
Galveston, TX 77550   Tel: (409) 761-1216

Application and Acceptance (1987–88):
Application made through the
University of Texas System, Medical and Dental Application Center, Suite 102, 210 West 6th Street, Austin, TX 78701
Application filing: April 15–Oct. 15, 1986
Application Center fees
Resident: $35 (plus $5 for each additional school applied to in the University of Texas system)
Nonresident: $70 (plus $10 for each additional school applied to in the University of Texas system)
Notification from: Jan. 15, 1987
Estimated new entrants: 203
School starts: Aug. 1987

Approximate Expenses per Year (1985–86):
Tuition: $400 (resident); $1,200 (nonresident)
Fees: $600
Other costs: $9,000

Statistics (1985–86):
Applicants: 2,342 (1,732 in-state; 610 out-of-state)
New entrants: 203 (185 in-state; 18 out-of-state)
Average GPA: 3.47

Requirements: MCAT, 90 sem. hrs. of college credit (bachelor's degree recommended), preference given to Texas residents.

Required College Courses:	Years
Biology (1 yr. lab)	2
Inorganic chemistry (with lab)	1
Organic chemistry (with lab)	1
General physics (with lab)	1
Calculus	½
English	1

University of Texas Medical School at Houston

Office of Admissions—Room G-024
University of Texas
Medical School at Houston
P.O. Box 20708
Houston, TX 77225   Tel: (713) 792-4711

Application and Acceptance (1987–88):
Application made through the
>   University of Texas System, Medical and Dental Application Center, Suite 102, 210 West 6th Street, Austin, TX 78701

Application filing: April 15–Oct. 15, 1986
Application Center fees
>   Resident: $35 (plus $5 for each additional school applied to in the University of Texas system)
>   Nonresident: $70 (plus $10 for each additional school applied to in the University of Texas system)

Notification: Jan. 15–Feb. 15, 1987
Estimated new entrants: 200
School starts: Sept. 1987

Approximate Expenses per Year (1985–86):
Tuition: $300 (resident); $900 (nonresident)
Fees: $300
Other costs: $7,600

Statistics (1985–86):
Applicants: 2,436 (1,729 in-state; 707 out-of-state)
New entrants: 201 (183 in-state; 18 out-of-state)
Mean GPA: 3.51
Sex: 39% women; 61% men

Requirements: MCAT, 90 sem. hrs. of college credit (bachelor's degree recommended), preference given to Texas residents.

Required College Courses:	Years
Biology (1 yr. lab)	2
Inorganic chemistry (with lab)	1
Organic chemistry (with lab)	1
Physics (with lab)	1
Calculus	½
English	1

University of Texas Medical School at San Antonio

Betty M. Compton
Registrar
University of Texas
Medical School at San Antonio
7703 Floyd Curl Drive
San Antonio, TX 78284   Tel: (512) 691-6906

Application and Acceptance (1987–88):
Application made through the
    University of Texas System, Medical and Dental Application Center, Suite 102, 210 West 6th Street, Austin, TX 78701
Application filing: April 15–Oct. 15, 1986
Application Center fees
    Resident: $35 (plus $5 for each additional school applied to in the University of Texas system)
    Nonresident: $70 (plus $10 for each additional school applied to in the University of Texas system)
Notification from: Jan. 15, 1987
Estimated new entrants: 202
School starts: Aug. 1987

Approximate Expenses per Year (1985–86):
Tuition: $300 (resident); $900 (nonresident)
Fees: $700
Other costs: $10,800

Statistics (1985–86):
Applicants: 2,298 (1,721 in-state; 577 out-of-state)
New entrants: 202 (184 in-state; 18 out-of-state)
Mean GPA: 3.45
Sex: 30% women; 70% men

Requirements: MCAT, three years of college (90 sem. hrs.), preference given to Texas residents.

Required College Courses: Years
Biology (1 yr. lab)..2
Inorganic chemistry (with lab) 1
Organic chemistry (with lab) 1
General physics (with lab) 1
Calculus ....½
English...1

University of Utah School of Medicine

Admissions Office
University of Utah
School of Medicine
50 North Medical Drive
Salt Lake City, UT 84132   Tel: (801) 581-7498

Application and Acceptance (1987–88):
AMCAS application filing: June 15–Oct. 15, 1986
Fee: $25
Offers Early Decision Plan (under which nonresidents must apply)
    EDP application filing: June 15–Aug. 1, 1986
    Notification by: Oct. 1, 1986
Regular applicants notified: Oct. 15, 1986–March 15, 1987
Deposit: $100
Estimated new entrants: 100
School starts: Sept. 1987

Approximate Expenses per Year (1985–86):
Tuition: $3,400 (resident); $7,400 (nonresident)
Fees: $300
Other costs: $4,400

Statistics (1985–86):
Applicants: 606 (257 in-state; 349 out-of-state)
New entrants: 100 (77 in-state; 23 out-of-state)

Requirements: MCAT, bachelor's degree recommended, prefer-
    ence given to Utah residents and WICHE-certified resi-
    dents of Idaho and Wyoming.

Required College Courses: Years
Chemistry (incl. inorganic and organic, qualitative and
    quantitative analysis; lab)..2
General physics (incl. heat, light, electricity, magnetism; lab)....1
English (composition and/or basic communication)....................1
Biology
Humanities
Social sciences

University of Vermont College of Medicine

Admissions Office
University of Vermont
College of Medicine
Burlington, VT 05405   Tel: (802) 656-2154

Application and Acceptance (1987–88):
AMCAS application filing: June 15–Nov. 1, 1986
Fee: $25
Notification from: late Dec. 1986
Deposit: $100
Estimated new entrants: 93
School starts: Aug. 1987

Approximate Expenses per Year (1985–86):
Tuition: $7,000 (resident); $9,300 (Maine); $7,000 (Rhode Island); $13,400 (New York); $16,000 (other states)
Fees: $300
Other costs: $7,300

Statistics (1985–86):
Applicants: 2,539 (83 in-state; 2,456 out-of-state)
New entrants: 93 (35 in-state; 58 out-of-state)
Mean GPA: 3.39
Sex: 39% women; 61% men

Requirements: MCAT, three years of college (bachelor's degree recommended), preference given to residents of Vermont and the residents of the states of Maine, Rhode Island, and New York.

Required College Courses: Years
Biology (with lab) 1
General chemistry (with lab) 1
Organic chemistry (with lab) 1
General physics (with lab) 1

Eastern Virginia Medical School

Office of Admissions
Eastern Virginia Medical School
700 Olney Road
P.O. Box 1980
Norfolk, VA 23501   Tel: (804) 446-5812

Application and Acceptance (1987–88):
AMCAS application filing: June 15–Nov. 15, 1986
Fee: $50
Offers Early Decision Plan
    EDP application filing: June 15–Aug. 1, 1986
    Notification by: Oct. 1, 1986
Regular applicants notified from: Oct. 15, 1986
Deposit: $100
Estimated new entrants: 96
School starts: Aug. 1987

Approximate Expenses per Year (1985–86):
Tuition: $11,000 (resident); $16,000 (nonresident)
Fees: $500
Other costs: $9,600

Statistics (1985–86):
Applicants: 1,290 (642 in-state; 648 out-of-state)
New entrants: 96 (84 in-state; 12 out-of-state)

Requirements: MCAT, 100 sem. hrs. of college credit, prefer-
    ence given to residents of Virginia, with special consider-
    ation shown to residents of the Tidewater area of Virginia.

Required College Courses:	Years
Biology	1
Chemistry (incl. organic chemistry)	2
Physics	1

Virginia Commonwealth University
Medical College of Virginia
School of Medicine

Associate Dean, Admissions
Medical School Admissions
Virginia Commonwealth University
Medical College of Virginia
School of Medicine
Box 565, MCV Station
Richmond, VA 23298   Tel: (804) 786-9630

Application and Acceptance (1987–88):
AMCAS application filing: June 15–Nov. 15, 1986
Fee: $40
Offers Early Decision Plan
    EDP application filing: June 15–Aug. 1, 1986
    Notification by: Oct. 1, 1986
Regular applicants notified from: Oct. 15, 1986
Deposit: $100
Estimated new entrants: 168
School starts: Aug. 1987

Approximate Expenses per Year (1985–86):
Tuition: $4,200 (resident); $7,800 (nonresident)
Fees: $300
Other costs: $5,900

Statistics (1985–86):
Applicants: 2,621 (705 in-state; 1,916 out-of-state)
New entrants: 168 (126 in-state; 42 out-of-state)
Mean GPA: 3.47
Sex: 31% women; 69% men

Requirements: MCAT, 90 sem. hrs. of college credit, prefer-
    ence given to residents of Virginia.

Required College Courses: Sem.
Biology (with lab) 2
General chemistry (with lab) 2
Organic chemistry (with lab) 2
General physics (with lab) 2
Mathematics 2
English (from English Dept.)..2

University of Virginia School of Medicine

Office of the Dean, Admissions
Box 235
University of Virginia
School of Medicine
Charlottesville, VA 22908   Tel: (804) 924-5571

Application and Acceptance (1987–88):
AMCAS application filing: June 15–Nov. 15, 1986
Fee: $50
Offers Early Decision Plan
    EDP application filing: June 15–Aug. 1, 1986
    Notification by: Oct. 1, 1986
Regular applicants notified from: Oct. 15, 1986
Deposit: $100
Estimated new entrants: 139
School starts: Aug. 1987

Approximate Expenses per Year (1985–86):
Tuition: $5,200 (resident); $10,400 (nonresident)
Fees: $100
Other costs: $5,700

Statistics (1985–86):
Applicants: 2,701 (554 in-state; 2,147 out-of-state)
New entrants: 139 (99 in-state; 40 out-of-state)
Mean GPA: 3.47

Requirements: MCAT, 90 sem. hrs. of college credit (bachelor's degree usually required), preference given to residents of Virginia.

Required College Courses:	Years
Biology (with lab)	1
General chemistry (with lab)	1
Organic chemistry (with lab)	1
General physics (with lab)	1

University of Washington School of Medicine

Committee on Admissions
Office of the Dean, SC-64
A-320 Warren G. Magnuson
    Health Sciences Center
University of Washington
School of Medicine
Seattle, WA 98195   Tel: (206) 543-7212

Application and Acceptance (1987–88):
AMCAS application filing: June 15–Nov. 1, 1986
Fee: $35
Notification: Oct. 31, 1986–May 15, 1987, or class matriculation
    (Sept. 24, 1987)
Deposit: $50
Estimated new entrants: 175
School starts: Sept. 1987

Approximate Expenses per Year (1985–86):
Tuition and fees: $3,100 (resident); $7,800 (nonresident)
Other costs: $5,200

Statistics (1985–86):
Applicants: 1,736 (463 in-state; 1,273 out-of-state)
New entrants: 176
Mean GPA: 3.55

Requirements: MCAT, three years of college (bachelor's degree
    recommended), preference given to residents of Washing-
    ton, Alaska, Montana, and Idaho or, regardless of resi-
    dence, an M.D.-Ph.D. candidate, black American, Ameri-
    can Indian, or Chicano.

Required College Courses: Sem. hrs.
Biology 8
Chemistry (incl. 1 yr. organic; lab) 12
Physics 8
English
Mathematics

Marshall University School of Medicine

Admissions Office
Marshall University
School of Medicine
1542 Spring Valley Drive
Huntington, WV 25704   Tel: (304) 429-5500

Application and Acceptance (1987–88):
AMCAS application filing: June 15–Nov. 15, 1986
Fee: $10
Notification: varies
Estimated new entrants: 48
School starts: Aug. 1987

Approximate Expenses per Year (1985–86):
Tuition: $1,700 (resident); $4,300 (nonresident)
Fees: $300
Other costs: $7,500

Statistics (1985–86):
Applicants: 584 (218 in-state; 366 out-of-state)
New entrants: 48 (45 in-state; 3 out-of-state)
Mean GPA: 3.5
Sex: 40% women; 60% men

Requirements: MCAT, three years of college (bachelor's degree recommended), preference given to West Virginia residents.

Required College Courses: Years
Biology or zoology (with lab) 1
Inorganic chemistry (with lab) 1
Advanced chemistry (incl. min. 1 sem. organic; lab) 1
Physics (with lab) 1
English (composition and rhetoric) 1
Behavioral or social sciences 1

West Virginia University School of Medicine

Office of Admissions and Records
West Virginia University
School of Medicine
Medical Center
Morgantown, WV 26506   Tel: (304) 293-3521

Application and Acceptance (1987–88):
Application filing: June 1–Nov. 30, 1986
Fee: $10
Notification: varies
Deposit: $50
Estimated new entrants: 88
School starts: Aug. 1987

Approximate Expenses per Year (1985–86):
Tuition and fees: $2,100 (resident); $4,600 (nonresident)
Other costs: $4,900

Statistics (1985–86):
Applicants: 365 (243 in-state; 122 out-of-state)
New entrants: 88 (85 in-state; 3 out-of-state)
Mean GPA: 3.44
Sex: 25% women; 75% men

Requirements: MCAT, three years of college (90 sem. hrs.), bachelor's degree recommended, preference given to residents of West Virginia.

Required College Courses: Years
Biology or zoology (with lab) 1
Inorganic chemistry (with lab) 1
Organic chemistry (with lab) 1
General physics (with lab) 1
English (composition and rhetoric) 1
Behavioral or social sciences 1

Recommended College Courses: Calculus.

Medical College of Wisconsin

Director of Admissions and Registrar
Medical College of Wisconsin
8701 Watertown Plank Road
Milwaukee,. WI 53226   Tel: (414) 257-8246

Application and Acceptance (1987–88):
AMCAS application filing: June 15–Dec. 1, 1986
Fee: $45
Offers Early Decision Plan
    EDP application filing: June 15–Aug. 1, 1986
    Notification by: Oct. 1, 1986
Regular applicants notified: Nov. 9, 1986–Aug. 18, 1987
Deposit: $100
Estimated new entrants: 202
School starts: Aug. 1987

Approximate Expenses per Year (1985–86):
Tuition: $7,500 (resident); $15,000 (nonresident)
Fees: $100
Other costs: $8,400

Statistics (1985–86):
Applicants: 3,144 (484 in-state; 2,660 out-of-state)
New entrants: 200 (112 in-state; 88 out-of-state)
Mean GPA: 3.58 (residents); 3.6 (nonresidents)

Requirements: MCAT, three years of college (90 sem. hrs.),
    preference given to Wisconsin residents.

Required College Courses: Sem./Qtr.
Biology (with lab) 2/3
General chemistry (with lab)...2/3
Organic chemistry (with lab) 2/3
Physics (with lab) 2/3
English (composition) 2/3
Mathematics (algebra, analytical geometry)

Recommended College Courses: Arts, language, literature, his-
    tory, music, philosophy, social sciences.

University of Wisconsin Medical School

Admissions Committee
Medical Sciences Center, Room 1205
University of Wisconsin Medical School
1300 University Avenue
Madison, WI 53706   Tel: (608) 263-4925

Application and Acceptance (1987–88):
AMCAS application filing: June 15–Dec. 1, 1986
Fee: $20
Offers Early Decision Plan (residents only)
    EDP application filing: June 15–Aug. 1, 1986
    Notification by: Oct. 1, 1986
Regular applicants notified from: Nov. 15, 1986
Estimated new entrants: 155
School starts: Aug. 1987

Approximate Expenses per Year (1985–86):
Tuition: $6,100 (resident); $8,800 (nonresident)
Other costs: $4,000

Statistics (1985–86):
Applicants: 1,298 (455 in-state; 843 out-of-state)
New entrants: 155 (153 in-state; 2 out-of-state)

Requirements: MCAT, three years of college (90 sem. hrs.), bachelor's degree recommended, preference given to Wisconsin residents.

Required College Courses: Sem.
General and advanced zoology or biology (cell biology,
    comparative vertebrate anatomy, developmental
    biology, genetics; lab) 2
Inorganic chemistry (incl. qualitative analysis; lab) 2
Organic chemistry (incl. 1 sem. aliphatic and aromatic
    compounds; lab) 2
Quantitative analysis 1
General physics (with lab) 2
Mathematics (incl. algebra and trigonometry) 2

Recommended College Courses: English, biochemistry, calculus, humanities, social sciences.

Canadian Medical Schools

These listings provide you with capsule descriptions of Canada's sixteen medical schools, presented alphabetically by province. Schools in .the U.S. and Puerto Rico are listed beginning on page 175. Each entry opens with the school's name, address, and telephone number.

All but four of Canada's medical schools offer four-year programs. McMaster and Calgary are three-year schools, and Montreal and Saskatchewan provide five-year programs. For details about how to use this directory, turn to page 169.

Information for Applicants. U.S. applicants should be aware that Canadian medical schools admit very few U.S. students. Some do not accept any students from other countries at all. So think twice before applying and make sure you know the residency requirements. What's more, Canadian education, in general, is somewhat different from the U.S. Also, provinces in Canada follow varying standards. So pay close attention to these entries. You'll find that requirements in Canada are often markedly different from those for U.S. medical schools. Particularly noteworthy is the fact that Laval, Montreal, and Sherbrooke medical schools, in the province of Québec, offer all instruction in French. Consequently, at these three schools you must be fluent in French. All other Canadian schools offer instruction in English.

Eleven of Canada's medical schools require that you take the Medical College Admission Test (MCAT). For details, see page 80. Entries indicate whether the school requires the MCAT.

Applicants to medical schools in Ontario must apply through the Ontario Medical School Application Service (OMSAS). Completed forms and transcripts must be in the hands of OMSAS by November 15. You can obtain information and other documents by writing to:

OMSAS
Ontario Universities' Application Centre
P.O. Box 1328
Guelph, ON
Canada N1H 7P4.

For additional information about Canadian medical schools, write to:

Association of Canadian Medical Colleges,
Suite 1120
151 Slater Street
Ottawa, ON
Canada K1P 5N1.

University of Alberta Faculty of Medicine

Admissions Officer
2J2.11 Walter MacKenzie H.S. Centre
University of Alberta
Faculty of Medicine
Edmonton, AB
Canada, T6G 2R7   Tel: (403) 432-6350

Application and Acceptance (1987–88):
Application filing: July 1–Dec. 1, 1986
Fee: $24 (non-University of Alberta applicants)
Notification: July 1–Sept. 1, 1987
Deposit: $50
Estimated new entrants: 118
School starts: Aug. 1987

Approximate Expenses per Year (1985–86):
Tuition: $1,300 (Canadian); $1,900 (non-Canadian)
Fees: $100
Other costs: $6,500

Statistics (1985–86):
Applicants: 819 (427 in-province; 392 out-of-province)
New entrants: 119 (114 in-province; 5 out-of-province)

Requirements: MCAT, two years of college after senior matriculation, preference given to Alberta residents.

Required College Courses:
Biological sciences (general biology, genetics, vertebrate zoology, microbiology)
Chemistry (inorganic and organic)
General physics
Mathematics (calculus and statistics)
English
Liberal arts

University of Calgary Faculty of Medicine

Coordinator, Admissions and Student Affairs
Admissions Office
University of Calgary
Faculty of Medicine
3330 Hospital Drive, N.W.
Calgary, AB
Canada T2N 1N4   Tel: (403) 284-6849

Application and Acceptance (1987–88):
Application filing: July 1–Nov. 30, 1986
Fee: $15
Notification: April 30–Sept. 30, 1987
Deposit: $100
Estimated new entrants: 72
School starts: Sept. 1987

Approximate Expenses per Year (1985–86):
Tuition: $1,700
Fees: $100
Other costs: $8,500

Statistics (1985–86):
Applicants: 982 (342 in-province; 640 out-of-province)
New entrants: 72 (59 in-province; 13 out-of-province)

Requirements: MCAT, two years of college (bachelor's degree strongly recommended), preference given to Alberta residents.

Recommended College Courses: General biology, cell biology; mammalian physiology; organic and inorganic chemistry; biochemistry; English; physics; calculus; one course of psychology, sociology, or anthropology.

University of British Columbia Faculty of Medicine

Office of the Dean, Faculty of Medicine
Admissions Office
University of British Columbia
2194 Health Sciences Mall, University Campus
Vancouver, BC
Canada V6T 1W5   Tel: (604) 228-4482

Application and Acceptance (1987–88):
Application filing: Aug. 15, 1986–Jan. 15, 1987
Fee: $25 (out-of-province applicants)
Notification: Jan. (approx.)–Sept. 3, 1987
Deposit: $100
Estimated new entrants: 130
School starts: Sept. 1987

Approximate Expenses per Year (1985–86):
Tuition: $2,500
Fees: $100
Other costs: $8,300

Statistics (1985–86):
Applicants: 577 (477 in-province; 100 out-of-province)
New entrants: 130 (130 in-province; 0 out-of-province)

Requirements: MCAT, three years of college (90 sem. hrs.),
minimum B average, preference given to British Columbia
residents.

Required College Courses: Years
General biology 1
General physics 1
General biochemistry or cell biology 1
General chemistry 1
Organic chemistry 1
Calculus I and II 1
English (literature and composition) 1

Recommended College Courses: Humanities, behavioral sciences.

University of Manitoba Faculty of Medicine

Director of Admissions
University of Manitoba
Winnipeg, MB
Canada R3T 2N2   Tel: (204) 474-8343

Application and Acceptance (1987–88):
Application filing: Nov. 1, 1986–Jan. 4, 1987
Fee: $25 (in-province); $50 (out-of-province)
Notification: June 1–June 15, 1987
Deposit: $100
Estimated new entrants: 95
School starts: Sept. 1987

Approximate Expenses per Year (1985–86):
Tuition: $1,400
Fees: $100
Other costs: $7,000

Statistics (1985–86):
Applicants: 249 (228 in-province; 21 out-of-province)
New entrants: 95 (95 in-province; 0 out-of-province)
Mean GPA: minimum 3.5

Requirements: MCAT, two years of college after senior matriculation, preference given to undergraduates and graduates of
the universities in Manitoba who are Canadian citizens.

Required College Courses:	Years
Biology (with lab)	1
Inorganic chemistry	1
Organic chemistry	1
Biochemistry	1
General physics	1
English	1

Memorial University of Newfoundland Faculty of Medicine

Chairman
Committee on Admissions
Memorial University of Newfoundland
Faculty of Medicine
St. John's, NF
Canada A1B 3V6   Tel: (709) 737-6615

Application and Acceptance (1987–88):
Application filing: Oct. 15, 1986–Jan. 15, 1987
Fee: $25
Notification from: April 25, 1987
Deposit: $100
Estimated new entrants: 56
School starts: Sept. 1987

Approximate Expenses per Year (1985–86):
Tuition: $1,000
Fees: $100
Other costs: $5,200

Statistics (1985–86):
Applicants: 607 (146 in-province; 461 out-of-province)
New entrants: 56 (40 in-province; 16 out-of-province)

Requirements: MCAT, two years of college, preference given to residents of Newfoundland and Labrador, New Brunswick, and the Maritime Provinces.

Required College Courses: Sem.
General chemistry 2
Organic chemistry (2nd-yr. level) 2
Mathematics 2
English 2

Recommended College Courses: Biology, physical chemistry, physics, behavioral sciences.

Dalhousie University Faculty of Medicine

Admissions Office
15th Floor, Sir Charles Tupper Medical Building
Dalhousie University
Halifax, NS
Canada B3H 4H7   Tel: (902) 424-3591; 424-7068

Application and Acceptance (1987–88):
Application filing: Oct. 1–Dec. 15, 1986
Fee: $15
Notification: Feb.–Sept. 1987
Deposit: $100
Estimated new entrants: 96
School starts: Sept. 1987

Approximate Expenses per Year (1985–86):
Tuition: $1,900 (Canadian); $3,300 (non-Canadian)
Fees: $100
Other costs: $6,000

Statistics (1985–86):
Applicants: 415 (232 in-province; 183 out-of-province)
New entrants: 96 (87 in-province; 9 out-of-province)

Requirements: MCAT, bachelor's degree, valid first-aid certifi-
cate from St. John Ambulance, preference given to residents of the Maritime Provinces.

Required College Courses: Sem.
General biology 2
General or inorganic chemistry 2
Organic chemistry 2
General physics 2
English 2

McMaster University School of Medicine

Assistant Registrar (Health Sciences)
Room 1B7, Health Sciences Center
McMaster University
1200 Main Street West
Hamilton, ON
Canada L8N 3Z5   Tel: (416) 525-9140, Ext. 2114

Application and Acceptance (1987–88):
Application made through the
    Ontario Medical School Application
      Service (OMSAS)
    Ontario Universities' Application Centre
    P.O. Box 1328
    Guelph, Ontario
    Canada N1H 7P4
OMSAS application filing: July 1–Nov. 15, 1986
OMSAS fee: $13
Notification: May 31–July 13, 1987
Estimated new entrants: 100
School starts: Sept. 1987

Approximate Expenses per Year (1985–86):
Tuition: $2,100 (Canadian); $3,200 (non-Canadian)
Other costs: $10,000

Statistics (1985–86):
Applicants: 2,800 (2,200 in-province; 600 out-of-province)
New entrants: 100 (96 in-province; 4 out-of-province)

Requirements: Three years of college, minimum B average,
    preference given to Canadian citizens or landed immigrants
    of the Hamilton health region and Northwestern Ontario.

Required College Courses: No specific course requirements.

University of Ottawa School of Medicine

Admissions, Faculty of Health Sciences
University of Ottawa
School of Medicine
451 Smythe Road
Ottawa, ON
Canada K1H 8M5   Tel: (613) 737-6463

Application and Acceptance (1987–88):
Application made through the
    Ontario Medical School Application
       Service (OMSAS)
    Ontario Universities' Application Centre
    P.O. Box 1328
    Guelph, Ontario
OMSAS application filing: July 15–Nov. 15, 1986
OMSAS fee: $13
Notification: May–Aug. 1987
Deposit: $100
Estimated new entrants: 84
School starts: Sept. 1987

Approximate Expenses per Year (1985–86):
Tuition: $1,600 (Canadian); $7,500 (non-Canadian)
Fees: $200
Other costs: $7,000

Statistics (1985–86):
Applicants: 2,133 (1,608 in-province; 525 out-of-province)
New entrants: 82 (75 in-province; 7 out-of-province)
Mean GPA: minimum B+

Requirements: MCAT, two years of college, Canadian citizen or
    landed immigrant.

Required College Courses: Years
General biology or zoology 1
General or inorganic chemistry 1
Organic chemistry 1
Physics 1

Queen's University Faculty of Medicine

Admissions Office
Queen's University
Faculty of Medicine
Kingston, ON
Canada K7L 3N6   Tel: (613) 547-5967

Application and Acceptance (1987–88):
Application made through the
    Ontario Medical School Application
      Service (OMSAS)
    Ontario Universities' Application Centre
    P.O. Box 1328
    Guelph, Ontario
    Canada N1H 7P4
OMSAS application filing: July 1–Nov. 15, 1986
OMSAS fee: $14
Notification from: May 31, 1987
Estimated new entrants: 75
School starts: Sept. 1987

Approximate Expenses per Year (1985–86):
Tuition: $1,500 (Canadian); $6,200 (non-Canadian)
Fees: $200
Other costs: $6,000

Statistics (1985–86):
Applicants: 2,410 (1,757 in-province; 653 out-of-province)
New entrants: 72 (56 in-province; 16 out-of-province)

Requirements: MCAT, two years of university beyond Grade
    XIII, Canadian citizenship or landed immigrant status.

Required College Courses:	Courses
General biology (with lab)	1
General or inorganic chemistry (with lab)	1
Organic chemistry (with lab)	1
General physics (with lab)	1

University of Toronto Faculty of Medicine

Admissions Officer
University of Toronto
Faculty of Medicine
Toronto, ON
Canada M5S 1A8   Tel: (416) 978-2717

Application and Acceptance (1987–88):
Application made through the
   Ontario Medical School Application
     Service (OMSAS)
   Ontario Universities' Application Centre
   P.O. Box 1328
   Guelph, Ontario
   Canada N1H 7P4
OMSAS application filing: July 1–Nov. 1, 1986
OMSAS fee: $14
Notification from: May 1987
Estimated new entrants: 252
School starts: Sept. 1987

Approximate Expenses per Year (1985–86):
Tuition: $1,600 (Canadian); $7,500 (non-Canadian)
Fees: $300
Other costs: $7,000

Statistics (1985–86):
Applicants: 2,401 (1,769 in-province; 632 out-of-province)
New entrants: 250 (232 in-province; 18 out-of-province)

Requirements: MCAT, Grade XIII plus two years of college (in
   a Canadian university) or Grade XII plus four years of college
   (in a non-Canadian university), bachelor's degree required
   for premedical studies taken in a university outside of
   Canada, preference given to Ontario residents.

Required College Courses: Years
Biology or zoology (Grade XIII, Level 5, or university
   level; lab) 1
General chemistry (quantitative or qualitative analysis,
   physical chemistry; lab) 1
Organic chemistry (with lab) 1
Physics (Grade XIII, Level 5, or university level; lab) 1

Statistics or biometrics (university level) must be completed
prior to enrollment in the second medical year.

University of Western Ontario Faculty of Medicine

Associate Registrar, Admissions
Stevenson–Lawson Building
University of Western Ontario
London, ON
Canada N6A 5B8   Tel: (519) 679-6530

Application and Acceptance (1987–88):
Application made through the
  Ontario Medical School Application
    Service (OMSAS)
  Ontario Universities' Application Centre
  P.O. Box 1328
  Guelph, Ontario
  Canada N1H 7P4
OMSAS application filing: July 1–Nov. 15, 1986
OMSAS fee: $14
Notification: May–early Sept. 1987
Estimated new entrants: 105
School starts: Sept. 1987

Approximate Expenses per Year (1985–86):
Tuition: $1,800 (Canadian); $6,900 (non-Canadian)
Other costs: $5,500

Statistics (1985–86):
Applicants: 1,987 (1,673 in-province; 314 out-of-province)
New entrants: 105 (103 in-province; 2 out-of-province)
Mean GPA: minimum 3.6

Requirements: MCAT, Grade XIII plus two years of college, Canadian citizenship or landed immigrant status, preference given to residents of Ontario.

Required College Courses:	Years
Biology (with lab)	1
Chemistry (incl. organic; lab)	1
General physics (with lab)	1
Arts and/or social sciences	2

Recommended College Courses: Behavioral science.

Laval University Faculty of Medicine

Secretary, Admissions Committee
Laval University
Faculty of Medicine
Ste.-Foy, PQ
Canada, G1K 7P4   Tel: (418) 656-2492

Application and Acceptance (1987–88):
Application filing: Dec. 1, 1986–March 1, 1987
Fee: $15
Notification from: May 15, 1987
Estimated new entrants: 150
School starts: Sept. 1987

Approximate Expenses per Year (1985–86):
Tuition: $700 (Canadian); $4,400 (non-Canadian)
Fees: $100
Other costs: $5,300

Statistics (1985–86):
Applicants: 1,324 (1,252 in-province; 72 out-of-province)
New entrants: 160 (152 in-province; 8 out-of-province)

Requirements: Fluency in the French language; two years of
college (Health Sciences Program) and the diploma of collegial studies of the Ministry of Education (Québec), or
equivalent; preference given to residents of the province of
Québec.

Required College Courses: Sem. hrs.
General biology (with lab)...8
General or inorganic chemistry (with lab) 8
Organic chemistry 8
General physics (with lab)..12
Mathematics (incl. analytical geometry, algebra,
    trigonometry, calculus)...12
French
Humanities
Behavioral and social sciences

McGill University Faculty of Medicine

Admissions Office
McGill University
Faculty of Medicine
3655 Drummond Street
Montreal, PQ
Canada H3G 1Y6   Tel: (514) 392-4232

Application and Acceptance (1987–88):
Application filing: Aug. 1, 1986–Dec. 1, 1986 (out-of-province);
    March 1, 1987 (Quebec residents)
Fee: $15
Notification from: March 15, 1987
Deposit: $100
Estimated new entrants: 160
School starts: Aug. 1987

Approximate Expenses per Year (1985–86):
Tuition: $800 (Canadian); $5,800 (non-Canadian)
Fees: $700
Other costs: $8,000

Statistics (1985–86):
Applicants: 1,420 (711 in-province; 709 out-of-province)
New entrants: 158 (105 in-province; 53 out-of-province)
Mean GPA: 3.7

Requirements: MCAT, applicants must be in the final year of
    their degree program, preference given to residents of the
    province of Québec.

Required College Courses:	Sem.
Cell and molecular biology	2
General chemistry	2
Organic chemistry	2
General physics	2

Recommended College Courses: Human and/or mammalian
    physiology.

University of Montreal Faculty of Medicine

Committee on Admissions
University of Montreal
Faculty of Medicine
P.O. Box 6207, Station A
Montreal, PQ
Canada H3C 3T7   Tel: (514) 343-6265

Application and Acceptance (1987–88):
Application filing: Dec. 1, 1986–March 1, 1987
Fee: $15
Notification: May 15–Aug. 1, 1987
Estimated new entrants: 160
School starts: Sept. 1987

Approximate Expenses per Year (1985–86):
Tuition: $740 (Canadian); $4,400 (non-Canadian)
Fees: $100
Other costs: $5,000

Statistics (1985–86):
Applicants: 2,028 (1,981 in-province; 47 out-of-province)
New entrants: 168 (163 in-province; 5 out-of-province)
Sex: 55% women; 45% men

Requirements: A thorough knowledge of the French language, two years of college (Sciences Program) and the diploma of collegial studies of the Department of Education (Québec), Canadian citizen or landed immigrant, preference given to francophone applicants from other provinces of Canada.

Required College Courses: Philosophy, behavioral and social sciences, French, English, mathematics (analytical geometry, calculus, algebra, trigonometry), sciences (biology, inorganic and organic chemistry, physics).

University of Sherbrooke Faculty of Medicine

Admissions Office
University of Sherbrooke
Faculty of Medicine
Sherbrooke, PQ
Canada J1H 5N4   Tel: (819) 565-5560

Application and Acceptance (1987–88):
Application filing: Nov. 1986–March 1, 1987
Fee: $15
Notification: April–June 1987
Deposit: $44.50
Estimated new entrants: 110
School starts: Sept. 1987

Approximate Expenses per Year (1985–86):
Tuition: $800 (Canadian); $4,400 (non-Canadian)
Fees: $200
Other costs: $5,000

Statistics (1985–86):
Applicants: 1,498 (1,450 in-province; 48 out-of-province)
New entrants: 110 (107 in-province; 3 out-of-province)

Requirements: Fluency and reading ability in the French language, two years of college under the present Québec educational system.

Required College Courses: Sem.
General biology (with lab)..2
General chemistry (with lab)..2
Organic chemistry (with lab)..2
General physics (with lab)..3
Mathematics (incl. analytical geometry, algebra,
    trigonometry, calculus)..3

Recommended College Courses: Humanities (incl. philosophy and literature), social and behavioral sciences (incl. history, psychology, sociology).

University of Saskatchewan College of Medicine

Admissions Secretary
University of Saskatchewan
College of Medicine
Saskatoon, SK
Canada S7N 0W0   Tel: (306) 966-6135

Application and Acceptance (1987–88):
Application filing: Sept. 15, 1986–Jan. 15, 1987
Fee: $25
Notification: June 1–June 30, 1987
Estimated new entrants: 60
School starts: Sept. 1987

Approximate Expenses per Year (1985–86):
Tuition: $1,500
Fees: $100
Other costs: $5,700

Statistics (1985–86):
Applicants: 271 (271 in-province; 0 out-of-province)
New entrants: 60 (60 in-province; 0 out-of-province)
Average GPA: 85.66%

Requirements: One full year of college work after senior matriculation (comparable with completion of U.S. college freshman year), Canadian citizenship or landed immigrant status, required to be bona fide resident of Saskatchewan.

Required College Courses:	Terms
Biology (with lab)	2
Chemistry (with lab)	2
Physics (with lab)	2
English (or another language)	2
Elective	2